The 10-20-30 Life Wellness Plan

A Manageable Plan to Instill Healthy Living into Your Life

Douglas C. Pearson

authorHOUSE®

AuthorHouse™
1663 Liberty Drive
Bloomington, IN 47403
www.authorhouse.com
Phone: 1-800-839-8640

The supportive reference material in this book is cited from some of the top experts in the field of nutrition, exercise, and health, but as with any health issue, this book is not intended to substitute for sound medical advice from your physician. The information in this book is not applicable to women who are pregnant. You should consult with a healthcare professional concerning any issues related to your health.

First published by AuthorHouse 1/18/2011

ISBN: 978-1-4490-7942-0 (sc)
ISBN: 978-1-4490-7943-7 (e)

Library of Congress Control Number: 2010918658

Printed in the United States of America

Certain stock imagery © Thinkstock.

This book is printed on acid-free paper.

Thank you to my family and friends who have supported and inspired me. May the rewards of a healthy lifestyle and the words in this book be an inspiration to others.

Table of Contents

Author's Note

"The health you enjoy is largely your choice."
—Abraham Lincoln

My interest in fitness, nutrition, and health traces back fifteen years. My lifestyle has always been an active one. I played sports in high school, maintained fitness in college as part of the Air Force Reserve Officer Training Corps, and passed all the fitness tests throughout my twenty-eight years in the U.S. Air Force. I still run, lift weights, swim, and bike. I teach wellness in school, and I am the head boys and girls' high school cross country coach, taking five teams to state meets over the past six years. From all this experience with health and fitness, the best lesson I have learned came about as a result of a routine annual physical while in the U.S. Air Force.

My desire to pursue wellness was a result of high cholesterol readings. In 1999, my total cholesterol was 236, and the unfavorable or bad LDL (low density lipoprotein) cholesterol was up to 162. I thought I had been living a healthy life, but now the doctors were concerned about my wellness. I was not overweight, and I was still very active. I found out that what you eat and the health choices you make—no matter what your age—do indeed make a difference in your overall wellness. What I learned and how I applied that knowledge are the basics included in this book. I developed and have lived *The 10-20-30 Life Wellness Plan* for the past twelve years, and I have maintained detailed lab records of my progress (see Appendix A).

I wrote *The 10-20-30 Life Wellness Plan* for young people and adults who struggle with many issues and the hectic pace of life today. My goal is to provide a compilation of key materials on life wellness in a condensed and easy-to-understand format. The book outlines a plan that addresses most of our health needs. *The 10-20-30 Life Wellness Plan*, used as a daily routine, will transform your behavior and become a lifetime habit of healthy living. The approach here is simple, yet it can yield positive results in preventing common medical problems associated with obesity, diabetes (Type II), heart disease, high cholesterol, high triglycerides, and elevated blood pressure.

I learned some valuable lessons from my experience with high cholesterol. I attended counseling sessions with a nutritionist, had repeated discussions on this topic with physicians, researched diets, and tracked my own experience in trying solutions so that I could avoid prescription drugs. The book summarizes the knowledge and experience I gained so that you can make proper health choices and live your life to its fullest. Knowing this plan works for me and could easily be followed as a lifestyle habit motivated me to share it with others.

My experiences with the negative impact of unhealthy lifestyles also provided the incentive for me to share this plan. My own high cholesterol was a personal motivating factor to improve my lifestyle. I know how family relationships can become strained when a person is dealing with obesity and associated health issues. I have seen how caring for loved ones, relatives, or friends can be difficult, especially when those last years are miserable because of poor lifestyle choices. I want to help and do something to make a positive difference in the lives of others. I want to motivate you to live a life of wellness!

"Our health always seems much more valuable after we lose it."
—Unknown

Introduction

"If we could give every individual the right amount of nourishment and exercise—not too little and not too much—we would have found the safest way to health."
—Hippocrates

This book is about wellness using a holistic and manageable plan. We all lead busy lives—going places, doing things, and constantly working to improve our lives. But consider too how unique we are compared to all other life on Earth. We can think, plan for the future, feel, and control many things that happen to us. We also can make choices that cause problems in our lives or make our lives better. Unlike other species on this planet, many humans have ruined their bodies through neglect, misuse, and indulgence in excesses that our lavish ways bring.

There are doctors who can prescribe medical solutions for health problems. There are counselors in nutrition who can advise you on proper eating habits. There are also experts in the field of fitness who can coach you on the best exercise regimens. All of these areas are important in providing you a complete wellness program. There are also diet books, recipe books, books on exercise regimens, and quick-fix solutions for every kind of weight and body image problem. Imagine the hundreds of books, all with solutions that work. The solutions, though, will only work if the individuals who buy the books follow the plans.

Even those with a solid education or background in wellness may find some of these books include complex plans too difficult to follow. Common sense indicates some of the published material may be too extensive for many people to apply to their daily lives. These books do offer solid advice and sound methods, and they are written by top experts in the field. In fact, many of them cover nearly 100 percent of what a person needs to do.

Part of the problem may be that the person becomes overwhelmed with the material and does not follow all the guidance. That's when the 100 percent becomes zero percent. The book is bought, reviewed, and read with the best intention of self-improvement. Then the method, the lack of motivation, or the complexity of the process takes its toll, and the book is put on the shelf, often in the company of many others just like it.

One reason why so many diet programs fail is that they require participants to track all of the food they eat—sugar, fat, salt, carbohydrates, serving sizes, calories, etc. The participant soon gets discouraged and stops the diet. *The 10-20-30 Life Wellness Plan* takes this into account. Simplicity in the approach is the reason this method will most likely work for you. My plan spells out how to live a life of wellness in areas you can control, simply and easily.

There has to be a solution that works—one that is easy to implement each day and motivates, one that is simple and meets the commonsense test. Common sense allows the plan of execution to be less than a 100 percent solution. A simple plan, even if it does not cover everything, is more likely to be understood, followed, and most importantly maintained as a lifestyle change. Someone following a plan that may only cover 80 percent of what you need to do is doing more than someone who gets discouraged from the start and does not follow a more comprehensive plan.

The 10-20-30 Life Wellness Plan is a nutrition and exercise regimen focused on developing and maintaining a healthy lifestyle. The plan is based on a simple, commonsense approach, and it is structured so it can become a normal daily routine that one can follow for the rest of his or her life. Each portion of this three-part plan is directed toward a specific health area, but the book still covers a broad range of wellness aspects.

The "10" in the chapter "Target the 10" refers to saturated fat grams. The plan requires that a person target and decrease their consumption to ten saturated fat grams per day. Most people eat many more than ten grams of saturated fat per day, but the goal should be to lower those saturated fat levels. This part of the plan focuses on avoiding the unhealthy foods. When a person concentrates on this portion of the plan and complies with the "10," many of these unhealthy foods will be eliminated from the diet.

The "20" in the chapter "Triumph over the 20" refers to fiber grams. The goal is to eat twenty grams of fiber or more a day. View the "20" as a baseline, and triumph over this minimum to achieve higher levels of fiber in your daily diet. When a person focuses on high-fiber foods, the daily meals will be dominated by more of the healthy foods.

The "10" and "20" parts of the plan simplify the nutritional complexity of counting calories, keeping track of serving sizes, monitoring consumption of multiple food groups, or calculating percentages of total calories for certain food groups. This plan allows a person to direct their attention to the two main components of nutrition. By following the "10," you will automatically exclude most of the bad foods from your diet. Following the "20" will help you incorporate all the good nutritional foods into your diet so that they can become part of your healthy eating habits. The best part of all this is that it will happen without you having to think much about it! You will find that you will become more saturated-fat-and-fiber conscious.

The "30" component of the plan outlined in the chapter "Thrive on the 30" involves exercise. The only way to maintain a long-term, healthy lifestyle is to incorporate a vigorous exercise plan into your lifestyle of wellness. You should thrive on thirty minutes of exercise a day. Individual goal setting is important to the success of establishing this portion of the plan so that you can develop a lifelong pattern. The exercise routines must alternate between demanding aerobic activity and weight-bearing workouts. The emphasis on exercise is paramount and significantly contributes to a healthy body.

The 10-20-30 Life Wellness Plan does not cover 100 percent of the solution, but it does provide practical applications to meet a majority of your wellness needs. I wanted to write this book to gather and sort through the maze of data out there and provide information that passed the commonsense test. Simplicity carries so much more meaning. It is an art to turn the complex into the simple, and it is the simple that is doable, understandable, and motivational.

This book brings together the expertise of others and blends their thoughts together with my life experiences as I struggled to get my cholesterol under control and found the will to change my life to attain better health and fitness. *The 10-20-30 Life Wellness Plan* is both a holistic and practical approach to enhancing health and well-being through nutrition and exercise. On the practical side, you will find simple, easy-to-follow exercise routines and assessment tools in the appendixes to help you get started. The book provides a commonsense, simple solution for a doable wellness plan that I hope will work for you just as it did for me. That is why I have such a strong passion to pass this information on to each of you.

"The problem with common sense is that it is not common."

—Mark Twain

On the Nature of Wellness

"If I knew I was going to live so long, I would have taken better care of myself."
—Mickey Mantle

As mentioned, the goal here is to make this simple. Behavioral science endorses the simple, commonsense solution with documented research supporting the importance of focusing on just three things. This is often referred to as "the power of three" and can be widely used in many areas of human behavior.[1] Brian Wansink, PhD, author of *Mindless Eating*, recommends focusing on just three areas as a way to make behavioral changes easier to assimilate into daily routines. This wellness plan uses the behavioral guidelines of the "power of three," focusing on three main components—the "10," the "20," and the "30." The plan is simple to understand and to follow, as its fundamental concept is summarized in just a few pages in the Introduction.

Understanding the three components of this plan does not result in improved wellness. No, a behavior change has to happen, and you must incorporate this wellness plan into your lifestyle. This simple plan will help you change your diet and exercise habits in a positive way, but your focus must be on behavioral changes in order to succeed.

"The power of three" may help here. I believe there are three things needed. One, you must understand and appreciate the uniqueness of yourself. You have the ability to make wise life choices, and when you do things right, do it with extra effort. Two, you need to become goal-oriented. Three, you must have a commitment to making your life the best it can be. It is all very simple. Applying it sometimes can be hard, but the rewards of a full, rich, and healthy life make the effort worthwhile.

This plan provided here is a total life wellness plan, more of a holistic approach, not just diet or exercise. Life wellness must address the whole person. It is not just a one-dimensional program; it's a life program. A good wellness plan promotes all aspects of human wellness. As a life program, it is important to focus on the holistic connectivity of all the categories of human wellness—nutrition and physical training, as they link together the functions of body, mind, soul, and spirit. Being a "life" wellness program means *The 10-20-30 Life Wellness Plan* is for everyone. The philosophy contained in the *The 10-20-30 Life Wellness Plan* is provided with the goal of making your life better.

You have a great deal of control to make your life the best it can be. Sometimes things in life do not go the way you want them to, but for the most part, the quality of your life is a result of your individual choices. The success in executing this wellness plan comes down to the choices you make and the behaviors you adopt for a healthier diet and better exercise habits.

How healthily you live your life is your choice. I want to give you the simple tools in this life wellness plan to make your life enjoyable and free of sickness in all areas you can control. I hope you apply this simple plan to your everyday living starting now. Hold on to this plan, because it is one that will work for you now, one you will be able to follow for the rest of your life. Also, share it with friends and family. It will work for everyone. It is not a diet, and it is not just an exercise routine. It is a pattern of living that ensures lifelong health benefits.

Status of the current lack of self-care in the United States

"The commonest form of malnutrition in the Western world is obesity."
—Mervyn Deitel

There is solid, substantiated medical proof linking poor self-care to health problems. Individual choice related to nutrition and exercise can go a long way in preventing many of the most common diseases currently impacting Americans. Excess weight is one of the more common self-care issues related to individual choices.

Of all the health problems associated with excess weight, the link to diabetes is the most impressive. There is now evidence that suggests we are in the midst of a growing international epidemic of diabetes. As weight increases, the risk of developing Type II diabetes rises dramatically. This has been a disease seen primarily in adults for many years, but now Type II diabetes has been diagnosed in more young people.[2]

Diabetes occurs when the body cannot make enough or properly use a hormone called insulin. Without this hormone, the blood sugar levels become elevated. High blood sugar levels result in impaired circulation, increasing the chances for heart attacks, strokes, kidney damage, nerve damage, and other health problems. Type II diabetes is a disease directly correlated to a person's individual wellness choices. In extensive clinical studies, weight loss and regular exercise were shown to be more effective than the leading oral antidiabetes medication.[2]

To highlight the significance of this problem, the Centers for Disease Control (CDC) in 2004 announced: "America's weight problem is rapidly overtaking cigarette smoking as the leading cause of preventable death." If you are twenty-five pounds too heavy, you are three times more likely to develop coronary heart disease, two to six times more likely to develop high blood pressure, and three times as likely to get Type II diabetes.

Heavier people also have a higher risk for cancer. Of course, all of this traces back to choices you make. The foods we eat, the amount of exercise we get, the hygiene we practice, the stress we undergo, and the unbalanced lives we lead account for about 65 percent of cancer deaths in the United States.[3]

It is important to focus on health issues related to the lack of personal wellness and the extent of this problem. The following compilation of statistics provides a sobering look at the impact of so many poor individual choices made every day:

- One-third of those living in the United States are obese (thirty pounds overweight). Obesity creates health risks. Obese people have lifetime medical bills that range from $5,000 to $21,000 higher than their normal-weight peers.[4]
- We are raising a whole generation of young people who are not

healthy. Type II diabetes is now being seen in preteens. A child diagnosed with Type II diabetes as a preteen may have vision problems in their twenties, heart problems in their thirties, and kidney failure in their forties, and they may not even live past their fifties.[5]

- One in four American children is overweight. Research shows obese kids have lower self-esteem and more emotional stress than their normal-weight classmates. In one study, 80 percent of children who were overweight at ten to thirteen years old remained heavy as adults. There is a higher prevalence of atherosclerosis (blockage of the arteries) in younger people. Autopsies performed on teenagers show most between fifteen and nineteen had fatty streaks in their coronary arteries.[6]

- The CDC estimated 32 percent of children were overweight or obese, and that level has been steady since 1980.[7]

- Being overweight or obese, especially among children, has emerged as a serious threat to our nation's health. The number of overweight teens has tripled since 1980, and 65 percent of those twenty years old and older are overweight or obese. The problem of obesity in adults has increased 75 percent since 1991. Obesity disproportionately impacts African-American, Hispanic, and low-income groups.[8]

- Even though there is a solid connection between extra weight and many types of diseases, the statistics continue to show an increase in the number of overweight and obese people. In the United States, the rate has gone from 58 percent of the population in 2001 to 63 percent in 2005. Type II diabetes has also gone up from 7.9 percent to 8.5 percent in that time. All these changes took place in only four years.[9]

- In the last ten years, the prevalence of obesity has grown 34 percent. Now one out of three adults is obese. Obesity is defined as 20 percent over your desirable body weight.[10]

- We are the fattest nation on Earth, and we are increasing the obese population at an alarming rate. Two-thirds of Americans over twenty are overweight. The number of those extremely obese (at least a hundred pounds overweight) has quadrupled since the 1980s. Researchers at John Hopkins University predict that 75 percent of adults will be overweight (and 41 percent obese) by 2015. Dr. Youfa Wang, who led the study, stated, "Obesity is a public health crisis."[3]

The statistics above are extensive, and they highlight the consistent pattern related to poor health choices. To put this in perspective, consider how the health issues of Americans have changed over the past century. In 1900, the leading causes of death in the United States were pneumonia, influenza, tuberculosis and diarrhea. Heart disease was the fourth leading cause of death. Comparatively, from 1999 to 2004, the leading causes of death were heart disease, cancer, and stroke.[11]

The point here is that diseases of the past were not related to individual choices. These infectious diseases were not related to diet. As medical advances were made, vaccines and antibiotics helped control infectious diseases that caused problems for earlier generations. There were also advances in surgery and internal medicine that helped cure other illnesses. As a result, life expectancy increased in the more advanced countries.

Now the illnesses are centered on circulatory problems and cancer. The diseases that are the leading causes of death today are very different from the diseases of the past. We bring many of today's illnesses on ourselves because we do not eat right or get enough exercise. These are areas we can control, whereas in the past, we were often victim to diseases we could not control. It makes even more sense now to do what is needed to ensure that we stay healthy.

In today's society, diet and nutrition are gaining increased recognition for their importance in health and wellness. For example, it is now estimated one-third of cancer deaths are related to obesity and nutrition. Acknowledging the connection between diet, inflammation, and disease can give people a clearer picture concerning the power they have over their own wellness.[12]

This critical look at modern diseases from a nutrition and wellness perspective is important to understand. Health and wellness are more complicated medical problems than disease. With disease, the impact on the body is already observed and can be diagnosed. Once a disease is diagnosed and proper medical care is provided, the natural laws of physics take over. The healing process related to disease is an easier and simpler application of science than the preventive measures related to health or wellness.

With health or wellness, there is no problem to identify; however, the effort is to keep the body from getting sick. Preventive medicine is a challenge, because the science of all the mechanisms controlling the body is complex. Doctors must be able to understand the body and follow certain rules governed by nature.

Think of this like a train going down the tracks. If you have a disease and the train runs off the track, it is an identifiable problem with a clear fix. But to stay healthy and keep the train on the track requires knowing how the body works before anything goes wrong.[13] Many medical studies are now concentrating on the impact of proper nutrition, optimal levels of exercise, and overall wellness in reducing the risk of certain diseases—all areas that are individually controlled through proper health choices.

The statistics demonstrate the significance of the problem, but what is causing many Americans to become overweight? Some scientists argue our national obesity stems largely from our food choices. We choose to eat a calorically dense diet, one high in saturated fats, rich in sugar, and low in fiber and nutrients. We eat too much, and we eat the wrong things. In addition, we don't get enough exercise, especially strength-building exercise. All this has led us to classify more Americans as "overweight" than ever before.[14]

Eating too much fat may not be the entire cause of the problem. As with most problems, it could be a combination of factors. Most of the grains we eat are highly processed. The processing removes fiber and nutrients from the grains themselves. In 1970, the average North American ate about 135 pounds of grain. By 2000, that figure rose to nearly 200 pounds. Eating more grains without the fiber and nutrients has partially contributed to 61 percent of American adults being overweight and 25 percent being obese, which is double what it was twenty years ago.[15]

Scientific data clearly show a connection between what we eat, how we care for our body, and our overall life wellness. The link has been proven, connecting abdominal obesity as a risk factor for heart disease and that excess weight puts a strain on both the heart and lungs.[16] All the data and references cited connect high blood pressure, diabetes, heart disease, cancer, and stroke to individuals who are overweight.

Examining solutions to improve self-care

There is a solution to the problem of excess weight, poor nutrition, lack of exercise, and the associated impact on wellness. The purpose of this book is to "keep your train on the tracks" and help you maintain a lifetime of wellness. A lifelong solution is the best solution. There is no guarantee on living a life of wellness, because there are some factors we cannot control; however, we must take responsibility for the things that we can control.

There are no gimmicks, just good habits. The quality of your life is measured by the quality of your habits. Once you develop good habits, they will stick with you and become your lifestyle. What you look like, how you feel, and your overall health are cumulative effects of lifestyle habits. You only have one body to carry you through life, and if it is well cared for, your life will be much more fulfilling.

The wellness habits you develop will become more obvious as you age. Teenagers are not concerned about being thirty, forty, or fifty years old. Even young adults may not consider the future consequences of the health choices they make. Nonetheless, you should develop good wellness habits now so these behaviors become part of your lifestyle. At any age, if you realize you have not practiced good habits, you can always refer to *The 10-20-30 Life Wellness Plan*. It is so simple that you will remember it for the rest of your life, and you can adopt it at any time as a wellness routine.

Three areas of discussion are central topics in addressing solutions for improving wellness. The three things to focus on are commitment, nutrition, and exercise.[17]

This book is intended to help those who are looking for a positive change in their lives. You want a solution, and this wellness plan might be just what you need to take the next step toward a healthier lifestyle. The book's commonsense format will ease that challenge of making a commitment to eat better and get more exercise.

However, simple solutions do not always equate to effective results, because human behavior must "make it happen." The words "make it happen" are simple words, but they imply that you are in control. You can make the choice. You can take the solution and implement it. The words also carry deeper meaning—that it may not be easy to do. The first thing that has to happen for this solution to work is for you to make that initial commitment.

Making a commitment to eat better and get regular exercise must come from a deep desire within yourself to improve your chances for long-term health and happiness. It will take dedication, determination, and self-discipline. There will come times when you stray off the path to improved health and fitness, but if you keep at it and stay committed over time, the benefits you reap will be well worth the effort.

For example, did you know that about 70 percent of all serious illnesses are preventable?[18] The doctor's role remains a critical one, because preventive medicine is so much a part of what doctors must provide. But look at the huge role you play as well. Improved wellness can be a simple solution where the individual is engaged in his or her own preventive medicine by following a sensible life wellness plan.

How would you like to commit to something simple in life and live longer? This book is designed to provide you the tips and reasoning to guide you in the right direction so that you can live a healthier and longer life. You will not only add years to your life but add life to those years as well. The quality of your life as you live longer is greatly improved by following the ideas in this book.

In a study done by the University of Cambridge involving twenty thousand people, researchers determined some simple things can add years to your life. Researchers determined that not smoking, eating lots of fruits and vegetables (which contain fiber), and getting regular exercise can add as many as fourteen years to your life.[19]

Commitment implies doing something. It may be doing what you have been doing and sticking with it, but for many people, it will likely involve a behavior change to develop new and better habits. When behavior change is required, it helps to receive support from your friends and family.

But you still have to "make it happen," and nobody but you can motivate yourself to change. It is an internal drive, a type of work ethic, and a dedication to meet established goals. Studies have shown old habits can be replaced by good habits, and the behavioral changes will take hold if the new habit is maintained for twenty-eight days (about a month).[20] Give it a try and see what happens. Stick with it for a month and see if your new habits of wellness become a lifestyle of wellness.

Let's take a look now at how tough this challenge is and how hard it is to keep a commitment. Most of us know exercise is good for our bodies. Most of us know the basic foods for good nutrition and foods that are bad for us. People who struggle with being overweight may see the need for exercise and good nutrition, but they may also want a quick fix. There is no quick fix. Even trying to apply the simple *10-20-30 Life Wellness Plan* will not result in an instant remedy to an overweight or other self-care problem. The solution requires a long-term commitment and consistency in adopting good wellness habits.

Behaviors most resistant to change involve addictions. Poor eating habits can be a type of addiction. Of course it is not a chemical type of addiction, but overeating and trying to control food intake can be a very difficult problem to resolve. As Gordon Livingston, MD, stated in his book *Too Soon Old, Too Late Smart*:

> What is at work here is the psychological power of habit. The characteristics that render each of us unique are seldom the products of rational choice. Sometimes, of course, we choose to develop healthy practices. Regular exercise can be a life-enhancing routine. Our bad habits, however, tend to work their way into our life over time and become extremely resistant to change, even when they threaten to destroy our lives.[21]

What if I told you that something you were doing might cause you to die? Suppose you were ready to walk across a frozen lake. Analysis of that lake's ice shows it to be thick enough to only hold the weight of a medium dog. If an adult went out on the ice, the ice would break, and the person would fall into the frigid water. What percentage of people would still venture out on the ice and risk their life? I suspect the percentage would be very small. Most people would realize the risk is not worth it.

Now suppose you have lived your life in a very unhealthy way. You ate lots of food containing saturated fat, ate too much, gained weight, and did little to keep your body in shape. Over time, these habits took their toll on your body. Your cholesterol went up. Your triglyceride levels became elevated. Your blood pressure rose, and your arteries became blocked with plaque. You became a victim of coronary artery disease and a candidate for a heart attack. You are ready to walk out on the ice-covered lake even though you have been told of the dangers. What percentage of people would be willing to change their habits and live a life of wellness?

Research shows that more than 70 percent will still take that figurative walk out on the ice. Likewise, with self-care, over 70 percent will fail to make the changes necessary to improve their lifestyle.[22] Human behavioral change is the toughest part of this wellness plan. Only 30 percent who already know they may die early would actually implement *The 10-20-30 Life Wellness Plan* or any other solution.

Knowing what to do is only part of the problem, and all too often we fail to act even when we know what to do. Patients having near-death experiences or procedures performed to save their lives are asked to change their behavioral habits—a clear choice to change or die. With a clear understanding that blocked arteries (or a walk across an icy lake) will kill them if they don't change their lifestyle, change becomes the biggest obstacle to overcome.

Let's be realistic. Very few people will modify their behavior to improve their wellness. If only 30 percent of those facing death will change their habits, there will only be a small percentage of people who will make changes when not faced with a life-threatening health concern. With this method, however, you will learn this simple approach so that your chances of using these basic wellness principles and adopting a healthy lifestyle habit will increase.

The levels of commitment may vary as you go through different phases in your life and as you experience various situations. The solution, though, to enhancing and maintaining your wellness still rests with a lifetime focus on commitment, nutrition, and exercise— the fundamentals of *The 10-20-30 Life Wellness Plan*. Most people fail at achieving wellness because their motivation or commitment fails them, not because the wellness method is faulty.

You must motivate your mind to successfully change your behavior. Former Arkansas Governor Mike Huckabee, who lost over a hundred pounds, approached his self-care as a lifestyle change issue, the same approach used in the plan presented in this book. He said the following:

> For people who have tried other methods of diet or health management and none has worked, consider the approach that this is a life mission to adjust your eating habits and exercise routine. Do not approach this as how much weight you need to lose, rather approach this as a lifestyle change related to a health and fitness goal.[23]

Nutrition is an essential part of the total wellness package. There is a saying: "You are what you eat." It is important to understand some basics on nutrition in order to lead a healthy life. Many of the solutions related to nutrition are fads. There are numerous quick schemes to lose weight or solve your dietary problems. Some are good ones backed by science, research, and proven results. Other diets, however, may be marketed to sell their product—be it a pill, a program, or a magazine.

Examine these solutions with common sense and realize that most diets simply do not work. I have witnessed others who have tried diets that turned out not to be successful. I am sure you, too, are aware of diet failures, either personally or through someone you know. Research supports what we all intuitively realize—that 95 percent of diets fail.[24] Trying to set goals for weight loss usually is not the best idea.

The key to implementing proper nutrition is to establish a life wellness routine—a habit of eating right. The quick-fix weight loss plan will not become a lifestyle habit. Do not concentrate your effort on diets. Instead put your energy and commitment into a lifetime of daily exercise and sensible eating.

Ann Shattuck, a research nutritionist at the Fred Hutchison Cancer Center in Seattle, emphasizes the parental role when she says, "If you provide nutritious, low-fat, high-fiber foods and set a positive example, you can influence your kids' eating habits for the better." This statement relates directly to the "10" and the "20" in *The 10-20-30 Life Wellness Plan*. When you look at nutrition, take that simple approach—focus on fat and fiber. Kids under the age of two require a different diet and fat is important, but after that age, you do not require high-fat diets. Research shows kids will grow and develop just as well on low-fat diets as kids who eat fatty food.[25]

The biggest challenge and toughest change for most people is exercise. Yet exercise plays a major role in good health, and it is the key to living longer and maintaining a quality life as you age. With proper exercise and a lifetime habit of exercise, you can reduce the impact of the aging process. Think of exercise as a life-sustaining pill. There are no prescriptions required and no medical costs. Exercise is the secret to great health. You should exercise hard almost every day of your life. Exercise should include aerobics and strength training two days a week.[26] These recommendations relate to the "30" part of *The 10-20-30 Life Wellness Plan.*

The 10-20-30 Life Wellness Plan addresses most requirements for a life of wellness. It is not a 100 percent solution, and you do not need to apply it 100 percent of the time. The plan provides a framework for you to follow every day. Think of this in a similar way to what Pamela Peeke, MD, a noted fitness expert and author, states: "Consistency is crucial here. Those who do best stick with it consistently, day in and day out, remembering the 80/20 rule. Do it right 80 percent of the time, leaving 20 percent for just being human."[27]

Likewise *The 10-20-30 Life Wellness Plan* may only cover about 80 percent of what is actually required for a perfect wellness plan, but this plan has the essential mix of what you need to do, namely getting rid of the bad food in your diet by keeping the saturated fat intake low, bringing nutritious and healthy foods into your diet by increasing your fiber intake, and really focusing on exercise. The solution is that simple.

"Make everything as simple as possible, but not simpler."
—Albert Einstein

Your initial self-care assessment

It is important in any wellness plan to first assess your health. One way to measure your health is to evaluate your body fat. Excessive body fat can lead to many health complications, including an increased risk for diabetes and heart disease. There are many techniques to measure body fat, including scales measuring weight and the percentage of your body fat.

A common and widely accepted method to assess your body fat is the Body Mass Index (BMI). This is a measurement that assesses your body size by taking your height and weight into account. Several different formulas are available to calculate your BMI, but the one below is the easiest to use.

BMI = W (weight in pounds) ÷ H (height in inches)^2 * 705

According to the latest classifications from the American Heart Association, a BMI of less than 18.5 is considered underweight. BMI values of 18.5 to 24.9 are considered healthy. BMIs of 25.0 to less than 30.0 are considered overweight, and people in this range are at a higher risk of heart and blood vessel diseases. Obesity is defined as a BMI of 30.0 or more. These people are at an even higher risk of cardiovascular disease. Extreme obesity is defined as a BMI of 40 or greater. The table below is borrowed from the American Heart Association and provides an excellent classification for assessing your BMI.

Body Mass Index Table and Health Risk

Height	Minimal risk (BMI under 25)	Moderate risk (BMI 25-29.9) Overweight	High risk (BMI 30 and above) Obese
4 feet 10 inches	118 pounds or less	119-142 pounds	143 pounds or more
4 feet 11 inches	123 or less	124-147	148 or more
5 feet	127 or less	128-152	153 or more
5 feet 1 inch	131 or less	132-157	158 or more
5 feet 2 inches	135 or less	136-163	164 or more
5 feet 3 inches	140 or less	141-168	169 or more
5 feet 4 inches	144 or less	145-173	174 or more
5 feet 5 inches	149 or less	150-179	180 or more
5 feet 6 inches	154 or less	155-185	186 or more
5 feet 7 inches	158 or less	159-190	191 or more
5 feet 8 inches	163 or less	164-196	197 or more
5 feet 9 inches	168 or less	169-202	203 or more
5 feet 10 inches	173 or less	174-208	209 or more
5 feet 11 inches	178 or less	179-214	215 or more
6 feet	183 or less	184-220	221 or more
6 feet 1 inch	188 or less	189-226	227 or more
6 feet 2 inches	193 or less	194-232	233 or more
6 feet 3 inches	199 or less	200-239	240 or more
6 feet 4 inches	204 or less	205-245	246 or more

Another way to do a quick assessment of your body fat is the skin fold test. Grasp the skin on the back of your upper arm, halfway between your shoulder and elbow. Do not pinch any muscle, just the skin and fat. If the thickness of the mass is one inch (2.5 centimeters) or more, it is likely an indication of a high percentage of body fat.[28]

If you still want to try another test, the skin and fat on the upper thigh can also be checked. Sit in a chair with your feet flat on the floor. Use your thumb and index finger and gently pinch the top of your right thigh. Measure the thickness of the pinched skin with a ruler. If the skin thickness is three-fourths of an inch or less, you have about 14 percent body fat, which is ideal for a man, not to mention a very fit measurement for a woman, too. If it is an inch, you are likely closer to 18 percent body fat, which is a bit high for a man but desirable for a woman. If you pinch more than an inch, you have too much body fat, and you could be at risk for health issues related to excess body fat.[29]

Your body fat assessment is an important wellness factor. You should have a basic idea of your general body fat percentage as it relates to health categories (see Appendix B). Whatever your risk category, you still have a lifelong requirement to care for your body and do all that you can to promote your optimum wellness.

Goals and commitment to protect the uniqueness of you

Setting goals, being committed, and working hard to achieve those goals is essential to success in life. You must establish the lifestyle habit of becoming a goal-setting person. Make your goals measurable and attainable. Start with any goal, and just write it down. Maybe you want to just walk one mile two times a week for a month. You might set a goal of eating the "10" and "20" part of this plan one day a week for a month. Set any goal that improves your wellness. You have months and years to reset and continue to improve your goals. As a goal-setting person, you must have discipline. You must be committed, and you must be energized by the personal satisfaction when each goal is successfully met.

Why are you setting goals for yourself? Look at it as an investment in your future. As an adult, you can get a car and a home. You have possessions and appliances in the house, and you may even have a yard or a garden. You likely have worked hard to get an education, have financial assets, and may seek spiritual peace through the practice of your religion. How do you protect this life investment?

To protect those belongings, you buy insurance on the car and home. You change the oil in the car. You paint the house. You mow the lawn, and you take care of all your material assets. You get insurance on the possessions in the home. You take time to have an advisor manage your financial interests. You may devote time during the week to seek spiritual peace. You may even protect your family with various types of insurance in case you get sick or die. You use your education and apply it in your job to improve your financial status and lifestyle. You may even seek more education and invest more money and time to earn an advanced degree.

Why do a majority of people do all these things? These actions are done to ensure a better standard of living and protect your investments. Most people take care of all the tangible investments around them, but what about you? So many people put themselves last on the priority list. With investments, people often hear, "Pay yourself first." In your life, you must also put yourself at the top of the list. You are the most important asset in your life. Make the investment in you the top investment in your life.

Matthew Kelly, a noted author on living life with passion and purpose expressed his thoughts on setting goals and achieving victories in life in his book *The Rhythm of Life*. Kelly's words are well written and present many wellness goals in life. Included below is an excerpt from his book:

> We get caught up in certain patterns of behavior that are self-destructive, a rhythm of life that does not attend to our legitimate needs, a lifestyle that does not enrich and fulfill us. How do we escape these vicious cycles? Small victories are the key. If you decide to become a marathon runner, you don't go out and try to run a marathon straightaway. Many victories are won before a marathon runner's first race. Small victories, one upon another, are the making of every great champion.

Set goals that stretch you but do not break you. The habitual and repetitious achievement of such victories produces the quality of self-discipline in a person's character. If you give your body a choice, it will always take the easy way out. Your body lies. It tells you it cannot when it can. The body has a natural capacity to increase its strength and abilities. One thing is certain. If you do only what you feel like doing, your life will be miserable and you will be a failure.[30]

Incorporate the ideas from this section titled "On the Nature of Wellness" so that you can make your life the best it can be. Look at the health problems in the United States, and make it a goal to maintain your wellness. Be committed to your solution, and stay motivated to live a life of wellness through proper nutrition and exercise.

Think of the body you have. It is an amazing and complex form of life. Respect it, and treat it with dignity. You are a unique person. Each one of us is an individual, yet we share so many aspects of life with each other. We all have dreams and aspirations. We all desire to love and be loved. We seek truth and knowledge, and we have the courage to take on new challenges. We all value life for the miracle it is and all the beauty that surrounds us.

Earth is a most unique celestial body. Think of how rare it is to have all the beauty of life on a planet in this universe. Many believe that there could be life on other planets somewhere in the universe, but because the universe is so vast, many also believe that the distance between these planets that contain life could be at least two hundred light years apart under the best circumstances.[31] That means what they would see through their telescopes would actually be light that left the Earth over two hundred years ago. To their eyes, our civilization wouldn't yet have electricity, computers, cars, airplanes, and modern forms of communication. Even though we may not really be alone, we are for all practical purposes alone in the vastness of the universe. Planets with life are precious, and you are here in this spot in the universe. You are unique.

Think of how many things about the human body remain mysteries. Science continues to research the human body, making new discoveries that range from the abstract functioning of our thought processes to the detailed replication of cells. But there are many things we do know about, including how we can benefit from living healthy lives and how the body's basic needs can so simply be satisfied. Kelly addressed this topic in a most poignant way:

Our bodies are glorious creations and should be honored and respected. Regular exercise, a balanced diet, and regular sleep are three of the easiest ways to increase our passion, energy, and enthusiasm for life. They are among our simplest legitimate needs and contribute massively to the well-being of the whole person. Unless we attend to our legitimate needs in relation to the physical aspect of our being, our capacity in all other areas of our life will be reduced."[32]

You may also want to establish who you are from a more sacred perspective, or at least view yourself in a way that leaves you inspired. Consider the intricate and complex processes in which each part of our body interacts, integrated in such a way as to provide us a fully functional body. In his book *Quit Digging Your Grave with a Knife and Fork*, Mike Huckabee approaches the topic of our human body in this spiritual way:

Be a good steward of the body you have. Properly cared for, the human body is an amazing machine! All the senses—eyes, smell, touch, hearing, taste—surpass any machine ever made. Plus the human heart, circulation system, digestive system, brain and central nervous system all represent amazing systems that function flawlessly and in a multitask role. Whatever your beliefs, the human body is an amazing, fully functioning, living form.[33]

With the big picture now in mind, is it really too much to ask to do what we can to make our lives as healthy as possible through better diet and exercise? Living life to its fullest can best be accomplished by living life in this healthy way. Therefore, focus on your uniqueness, and gain an appreciation for who you are and how special you are. Treat yourself as that very special and unique person. All in all, take care of yourself!

"Your body is a temple, but only if you treat it as one."
—Astrid Alauda

Target the "10"

**"Our bodies are our gardens—
our wills are our gardeners."
—William Shakespeare**

The "10" I am referring to concerns saturated fat. Do not get this confused with total fat. There are good fats, but saturated fat is the bad fat. Eating too much saturated fat is like eating poison. Saturated fat and how your body handles it could eventually kill you. Nothing good comes from a diet high in saturated fat; however, it can be very difficult to completely avoid saturated fat. Because most people consume too much saturated fat, the effort should be to reduce saturated fat levels and target your intake to ten grams of saturated fat a day. Setting this level as a goal will help you become more saturated-fat conscious and eliminate some of the bad foods in your diet.

Think of how you take care of your car. You put quality gas in its tank. You change the oil routinely to keep the engine operating properly. Would you mix in some sand with your oil, or would you put water in with the gas? These combinations are sure to cause problems for your car. A car given the wrong fuels will not run properly. The human body is an amazing living machine, but like any form of life, it needs the right nutrients to function properly.

Of all the things we eat, why focus on saturated fat? Well, to keep things simple, efforts to reduce saturated fat provide an easy way to control your bad eating habits. First, you will have to start looking at food labels to see which foods have saturated fat in them. As you become more familiar with what you are eating (i.e., what fuel you are putting in your living machine), you will start to recognize the foods with high amounts of saturated fat. These are the foods you must cut back on or eliminate altogether. It is that simple. Foods high in saturated fat are not good for you.

If you follow this rule of "target the 10," you will be surprised how your eating habits will change. You will start to avoid bad foods. You will look for healthier foods and wisely select the foods you buy. If you eat out, you will begin to intelligently order your meals so that you can cut back on menu items with saturated fat. You will look for foods with more fiber. If you snack, you will start choosing more nutritious options. Your life will not change radically as soon as you start watching your saturated fat intake, but over time, your health and your wellness will improve. Remember that this is a life wellness plan, and your habits must change. Similarly, your behavior must change. You must do this for the rest of your life.

How much saturated fat is right?

There may not be any proven scientific answers concerning the right amounts and kinds of foods for you; however, you can still use *The 10-20-30 Life Wellness Plan* as a guide. Think of this book as a type of template to help you set goals. Even if you are close to these targets most of the time, you will still improve your health.

Experts on diet and nutrition recommend that you receive no more than 35 percent of your calories from fat. Figuring your fat intake requires the examination of food labels and the use of a calculator. The recommendation of consuming 35 percent of your calories from fat deals with total fat. Determining percent of calories from fat involves dividing the amount of the "calories from fat" that you have consumed by the amount of "total calories" that you have consumed and multiply by a hundred to get a percentage.[34]

The calculations are similar when you are focusing on saturated fat. The American Heart Association and the National Cholesterol Education Program have established a target threshold. They suggest that 7 percent of your daily calories should come from saturated fat. Other groups have suggested 10 percent or less. The American Heart Association also recommends levels below 7 percent of daily calories from saturated fat for those who have an LDL (low density lipoprotein) reading over a hundred or have coronary heart disease. Most people currently eat between 12 and 14 percent of daily calories as saturated fat. Anything less than that would be an improvement and provide greater health benefits.[35]

The following example illustrates the method used to calculate the recommended level of saturated fat:

1. Assume you eat 1,800 calories a day, and 7 percent can be saturated fat calories.
2. (1,800 calories) * (7 percent saturated fat) = 126 calories of saturated fat per day.
3. Note that one gram of fat equals nine calories.
4. Therefore, 126 ÷ 9 = 14 grams of saturated fat per day.

Using the same process, determine the actual amount of saturated fat consumed in a day.

1. First, assume you ate the same 1,800 calories, but you got 15 percent of those calories from saturated fat.
2. (1,800 calories) * (15 percent saturated fat) = 270 calories of saturated fat for that day.
3. Note that one gram of fat equals 9 calories.
4. Therefore, 270 ÷ 9 = 30 grams of saturated fat consumed for that day.

The above calculation is not one too many people perform every day. This method of calculating the amount of saturated fat requires knowing the total number of calories eaten in a day and the percentage of daily calories that come from saturated fat. Of course, it's not easy to determine these numbers on a daily basis. I also would bet that it is not a calculation too many people would perform every day for the rest of their lives. These are accurate methods of computing dietary consumption, but what you need is a simple, easy-to-apply technique.

It is logical to assume that many people may be getting fat just because this process of tracking dietary consumption is so difficult. We are all a bit lazy when it comes right down to it, and maybe even more so about our health. How can we apply all this information and make the process easier?

The recommended levels of saturated fat (in grams per day) cover an extremely narrow range. On the low end, 1,800-calorie intake in a day and 5 percent of daily calories from saturated fat equates to ten grams a day. On the high end, 2,500 calories a day at 7 percent of daily calories from saturated fat equals 19 grams a day.

Rather than the tedious calculations provided in the above examples, it is far easier to look at food labels and quickly count up the number of saturated fat grams you would otherwise consume each day. At 14 percent of daily calories consumed from saturated fat, most people are eating around 35 to 40 grams of saturated fat a day. To make the process easier and healthier, think of lowering the consumption of saturated fat from those higher levels to a target number of ten grams a day. This process is simple, and it provides a baseline number that is easy to target. By aiming for the low end, you are ensuring that you have a healthier diet. Keep it simple, because simple will work.

The functional fats that improve health

Fat can be good for you, too. In fact, the body needs a certain amount of fat to function. Fat provides energy storage and controls body temperature, and it is essential for cell development. Keep in mind that what you eat impacts your body at the cellular level as well.

Let's call these good fats "functional fats." The two types of functional fats are polyunsaturated and monounsaturated fats. The American Heart Association defines the polyunsaturated fats as "fats that have more than one double-bonded (unsaturated) carbon in the molecule." However, the monounsaturated fats have one double-bonded (unsaturated) carbon in the molecule. These fats are usually liquid at room temperature and remain liquid even when chilled. In comparison, the bad saturated fats have a chemical makeup with carbon atoms that are saturated with hydrogen atoms. Saturated fats are typically solid at room temperature. That said, the structure of these fats is important in the way the body uses them and builds its cells.

Naturally, it is important for your diet to have a balance of many nutrients, but do not think all fat is bad for you. The body functions best with the good, functional fats. The polyunsaturated fats include those omega-3s found in salmon, tuna, walnuts, flaxseeds, pumpkin seeds, and sunflower seeds. These fats help to clear your arteries and speed your metabolism. The monounsaturated fats are found in nuts, olives, corn, avocados, and olive and canola oils. The body has an amazing ability to take these fats, use them to burn other fats, help reduce cholesterol, and keep you feeling full.[36]

The body uses fats to carry certain vitamins, to make hormones, to provide a layer of insulation for maintaining body temperature, and to build the membranes that surround every cell in the body. These unsaturated fats are even used to produce testosterone, the hormone that leads to muscle growth.[36] Functional fats like omega-3s can also reduce blood clotting, regulate heart rhythm, stimulate the immune system, and minimize wrinkles.[37]

The foul fats that cause health problems

Saturated and trans fats are bad fats. Limit the saturated fats, and eliminate the trans fats. The trans fats are created in an industrial process that adds hydrogen to liquid vegetable oils, and this makes the product more solid. These trans fats are also known as partially hydrogenated oils. Let's call these bad fats "foul fats." You can identify them on the nutrition labels of any food.

It is very important to your health that you focus on these foul fats and do everything you can to control your intake of saturated and trans fats. How serious is this? Dr. Henry Lodge, author of *Younger Next Year*, stated that eating saturated fat can kill human beings when combined with a lifestyle of little exercise and sedentary living.[38] The medical results clearly point to a healthier, longer life by avoiding saturated and trans fats.

The body does not react favorably to these foul fats. Saturated fat has no place in diets that focus on health and proper nutrition. The Glycemic Index Diet is one such diet that emphasizes healthy eating with low amounts of saturated fat.[39] Saturated and trans fats activate the genes that increase the production of a specific protein. This protein in turn causes inflammation of the arteries.

What you eat can significantly impact biological processes in the body. Inflammation of the arteries is one of the major causes of aging. This type of inflammation, along with the other negative effects of a diet high in saturated fat, also contributes to the following health problems[39/40]:

- Reduced energy levels
- Loss of skin elasticity
- Heart disease
- Heart attack
- Stroke
- Type II diabetes
- Colon cancer
- Prostate cancer
- Breast cancer
- Ovarian cancer
- Compromised immune system
- Memory loss
- Alzheimer's disease
- Serious infections
- Arthritis
- Gallbladder disease
- High blood pressure
- Elevated cholesterol and triglyceride levels
- Gangrene
- Diseases associated with clogged arteries
- Plaque buildup along artery walls
- Cardiovascular disease

In one experiment, medical students were given a fatty meal to examine triglycerides. A special device was used to look at the small blood vessels in the eyes. Fat from the food entered the bloodstream and became visible when the fat clogged the observed vessels. Cells began to clump together and turn the blood into sludge even nine hours later. It is this process, which can be seen on a smaller scale in this simple experiment, that also occurs throughout the body and contributes to many of the diseases listed above.[41]

The impact of saturated fats on health was also verified by a twenty-five-year study that evaluated the development of coronary heart disease and the long-term risk of death. This study, cited in Michael Roizen's book *Real Age Makeover*, and others repeatedly show a strong correlation between the consumption of saturated fats and the development of cardiovascular disease. In addition, Michael Roizen, MD, cites that only 20 percent of cholesterol is absorbed from food. The other 80 percent is manufactured by the liver from saturated and trans fats.

Think of the process going on inside the body. You consume saturated fats, and the body produces plaque from these fats, which builds up on the artery walls. It is like pouring grease into the pipes in your house. The grease sticks to the sides of the pipes, and eventually water no longer flows down the drain smoothly. Likewise in the body, plaque buildup is stage one of cardiovascular disease and the resulting aging of the arteries. Saturated fat also contributes to the increase of LDL or bad cholesterol in the bloodstream. As Roizen cleverly stated, "Think of saturated fats with the 'S' in mind, meaning 'Stay Away.'"[42]

High intake of saturated fat contributes to obesity as well. Saturated fat is believed to increase the need for essential fatty acids, which in turn lead to the creation of excess body fat. Extra weight then leads to other health problems.[43]

The problem of gaining excess weight is a clear one from a scientific point of view. Every pound of fat stored on the body is equal to 3,500 calories. As fat is added to the body, more blood vessels are needed to nourish the added tissue. The added tissue creates a strain on the heart, which in turn can lead to high blood pressure. The higher blood pressure causes a strain on the vessels, stretching them and causing injury. Consequently, people who are overweight or obese statistically have a shorter life span.[44]

To motivate improvement in health, it is beneficial to understand how the body functions with the food it receives. Physiologically, there are many things happening in the body as it processes fat. What you eat and how it is processed impacts you on the cellular level.

Fat is important and provides the structure for all forty billion cells in our body, including the connections between our brain cells. Each cell that is created is built with fat, and we build twenty billion cells a year. The important thing to know about cell building is the beneficial role of the unsaturated fats, those functional fats. Functional fats provide the best ingredient in forming well-shaped and properly functioning cells.[45]

To fuel this cell building process, a natural diet is best. Healthy fats and oils come from olive, canola, soy, corn, sunflower, and vegetable oils. Other foods containing functional fats include nuts, fruits, vegetables, sardines, mackerel, and salmon.

Unfortunately, most of the fat that dominates our diets comes from saturated fat, those foul fats. Saturated fat creates an inflammation in the arteries, and the body recognizes that as a signal to decay. Obese and sedentary people are four to five times more likely to have inflammatory proteins in their blood. These proteins cause heart attacks, strokes, cancer, and even Alzheimer's disease.[45]

If your body does not have the functional fats to build cells properly, your body will then use the foul fats instead. Your cell walls will then be constructed using saturated fats. These ill-constructed cells will be a slightly different shape and generate local inflammation, which is linked to the diseases mentioned above.[45]

You can see that focusing on the "10" involves understanding functional fats, foul fats, and the impact each type of fat has on the body. Most importantly, though, you must become saturated-fat conscious. You must be aware that full-fat dairy products, including butter, cheese, milk, and cream, contain saturated fat. Most meat, especially sausage and bacon, is bad, too. You should also try to avoid fried food and eliminate trans fats.

Many of the diseases and illnesses related to nutrition are not concerns for most people—that is, until they get sick. It's important to know the facts about fats so you understand the necessity of developing a healthy lifestyle. Your choices influence your habits, and your habits establish your behavior. Once behavior is set, it is hard to change. Therefore, you should try to develop good behaviors now before you suffer the symptoms of an unhealthy lifestyle.

You have to make intelligent food selections. To make these smart choices, you need to know what is good for you and what is harmful. Some people do not have the information to make these choices regarding fat in their diets. Honestly, it took me half a lifetime to understand the importance of what we eat. The information on fats took a little longer for me to master. That is why this wellness plan focuses on basic, easy-to-understand information that can also be easily applied.

So keep it simple. Remember that the good fats—the functional fats—come from plants and fish. The bad fats—the foul fats—can kill you if they are consumed in excess. They come mostly from animal and full-fat dairy products. Keeping in mind the functional fats and the foul fats and knowing what is healthy for you will help guide you when you are making choices about proper foods. Use this knowledge to make the right choices concerning both types of fat and you will have fewer health problems, enjoy a healthier life, and live longer as well.

"When you acknowledge that you and only you are responsible and accountable for the choices you make, you have in your hands the blueprint for success."
—Lou Holtz

Triumph over the "20"

**"While we may not be able to control all that happens
to us, we can control what happens inside us."**
—Ben Franklin

The "20" in this chapter concerns fiber—fabulous fiber. Focusing on foods with fiber will help you include most of the good, nutritious foods in your diet. Though reducing your intake of saturated fat is the first step of *The 10-20-30 Life Wellness Plan*, the second step concerns your daily fiber intake, which should be no less than twenty grams per day and preferably much higher. If you buy and eat foods high in fiber and become more fiber conscious, you will undoubtedly start establishing and maintaining a healthier lifestyle.

Think of fiber as the Pac-Man in your body. It gobbles up the bad things in your blood and digestive track. Fiber also comes with nutrients to properly fuel your body. Physiologically, our body reacts in a very logical manner. Think of the body like a machine. Bad fuel (saturated and trans fat) clogs up the machine, but good fuel (fiber) keeps it running smoothly.

Combining twenty grams or more of fiber per day with a diet high in the functional fats discussed in the previous chapter will make the machine run even better. The body is a most complicated and amazing machine, and you can improve how it functions with proper nutrition.

Douglas C. Pearson

Recommendations on the amount of fiber

Most people do not get enough fiber. The average person, probably one who does not focus on fiber intake, consumes about seven to twelve grams of fiber a day. Fiber intake recommendations range from twenty-one to thirty-eight grams per day. Some of the specific recommendations for the amount of fiber you should consume each day are included below:

- The National Fiber Council, with its push for a high-fiber diet, recommends thirty-two grams of fiber a day.[46]
- The American Dietetic Association recommends that people consume twenty-five to thirty-five grams of fiber a day.[47]
- Annette Natow, PhD, advises men between nineteen and fifty years old should get thirty-eight grams of fiber a day, and those over fifty should get thirty grams. Women between nineteen and fifty years old should get twenty-five grams, and those females over fifty should get twenty-one grams.[48]

Eating thirty-eight grams of fiber a day is great, but this expectation may be largely unrealistic for most people. If you view twenty grams of fiber a day as your baseline and make attempts to "triumph over the 20," this would be a good compromise and definitely an improvement over consuming as little as seven grams, which is more typical.

Many people find it difficult to get these high amounts of fiber into their bodies in a day. This difficulty is easier to understand when examining people's basic knowledge about fiber. About 62 percent of people believe that meat is a source of fiber; however, there is not a single gram of fiber in meat. Fiber can only be obtained from plant products. Additionally, over 70 percent of people read food labels, but only 48 percent actually look at the amount of fiber per serving.[46]

Naturally, the above recommendations seem like lofty goals, but keep this process simple and manageable. Just focus on the fiber amounts on food labels and maintain a fiber-conscious attitude. You will find yourself buying different foods—foods with more grains, more whole wheat, more fruits, more vegetables, more oats, more nuts, and more high-fiber cereal. Your habits will change, and so will your health. This is not a hard habit to adopt, and it is one you can follow for the rest of your life. Remember that habits change behaviors, and behaviors change lifestyles. You are on a mission to live a healthy lifestyle, and this wellness plan is your road map.

Fabulous fiber—types and benefits

There are two basic types of fiber: soluble and insoluble fiber. Soluble fibers dissolve in water and form a gel-like consistency. Oat bran, grains, legumes (peas and beans), carrots, oranges, nuts, barley, flaxseed, apple, and citrus pectin all contain soluble fiber. This type of fiber has been shown to help lower cholesterol levels by pulling cholesterol from the bloodstream. Soluble fiber also slows digestion, which allows you lasting energy.[49]

The other type of fiber is insoluble fiber. This fiber does not dissolve in water. Vegetable and fruit skins, green beans, dark leafy vegetables, whole wheat products like wheat bran and whole grains, corn bran, seeds, and nuts all deliver insoluble fiber. Medical studies indicate insoluble fiber seems to reduce the risk of cancer.

Insoluble fiber acts like the Pac-Man referenced earlier. It rapidly travels through the body, and as it goes through your plumbing system, it picks up miscellaneous fats and whatever else is lingering around. Fiber is not digested; it simply passes through the body. Fiber does not get absorbed into the bloodstream, but it does have a positive impact on blood chemistry. It works like a flushing action and ushers all the unfavorable things in your system out of your body.[49]

There is no need to complicate things here by trying to count the grams of soluble fiber and insoluble fiber you consume. The purpose here is to provide a plan that involves tracking two basic nutrition components, namely saturated fat and total fiber. The plan is more likely to be successful if it is easy to follow and easy to achieve. Just "triumph over the 20," and you will get a good enough mix of both fibers to improve your health.

All the studies and research on nutrition indicate that fiber is very beneficial to the body and contributes to a healthy lifestyle. Plant foods are high in fiber, but animal foods do not contain any fiber. This does not mean you should avoid meat, but your diet should be rich in fruits, vegetables, nuts, berries, whole grains, beans, and any plant-based food.

Lists are good. They present lots of information in a simple way. Here is a list of all the benefits of fiber:[50/51/52]

- Fiber aids in digestion.
- Fiber binds with cholesterol and carries it out of the body.
- Fiber helps balance glucose levels in the blood.
- Some fibers bind to cancer-causing agents in the digestive track and sweep them out of the body.
- Fiber helps prevent the accumulation of body fat, because it is hard to eat a diet high in fiber and also gain weight.
- Fiber helps fight diseases.
- Most high-fiber foods contain certain chemicals with anticancer effects.
- Dietary fiber may help prevent appendicitis.
- Fiber provides a low-calorie filler, slows the digestive process, and makes you feel satiated.

Many references support the fact that fiber is a powerfully medicinal food.[53/54] The health benefits of a high-fiber diet are reduced risk of heart disease, artery disease, gall bladder disease, and cancer (colon, bladder, breast, cervical, and lung). Fiber also provides better control of existing diabetes by stabilizing glucose levels in the blood. A high-fiber diet has also been linked to a lower risk of diabetes, especially when combined with weight loss and exercise. Diets high in fiber have been shown to help individuals shed excess body fat and combat obesity. Fiber may also help lower blood pressure by about 10 percent.

Natural foods are rich with fiber. The problem, however, is that many of the foods we eat now are processed beyond their natural state. Consequently, the body will do less work during digestion when these processed foods are consumed. In his book *Living the Glycemic Index Diet*, Rick Galloop provides an excellent source of recipes for meals with high fiber and healthy eating.[52] He states that the fundamental problem is that the foods we eat are digested too easily by our bodies. Foods lose much of their inherent nutritional value and health benefit when they are processed. The fiber in foods is lost in the processing, and fiber is the source of so many health benefits.

The benefits of fiber lead to improved health and a longer lifespan. By eating the right foods, you provide nourishment to your body. When properly fueled, the body functions at its best. Michael Roizen, MD, examined the impact of fiber consumption on longevity. His results show that if people eat more fiber, they can significantly lower their rate of aging. A Northwestern University study determined a ten-gram increase in daily fiber from cereal decreased the risk of heart attack by 29 percent. If your eating habits do not involve adequate fiber, you are much more likely to have a poor diet and become more sedentary.[55]

Examination of food pyramids and summary of nutrition

The information in "Target the 10" and "Triumph over the 20" provides guidance on healthy eating. Obviously, what you put in your body makes a difference. The latest research suggests that inflammation of the arteries may create as big a risk for heart disease as clogging of the arteries because of cholesterol deposits. A high-fiber diet with plenty of beneficial fats proved better at controlling damaging inflammation than the standard low-fat diet. In a two-year clinical trial, medical experts confirmed the health benefits of combining a diet high in fiber with functional fats.[56]

This clinical trial is just another reference that illustrates the overall importance of the combined "10" and "20" approach. Developing a habit of eating the right foods the majority of the time will change your health profile. It is simple—*Eat plenty of fiber and good fat, and avoid the bad fat.* The health benefits of this method of eating are well documented. I have listed the health benefits of fabulous fiber, detailed how the body performs better with functional fats, and listed the health problems associated with foul fats. In addition, I have developed this simple nutritional advice based on reference material from many of the top medical and diet experts.

The food pyramid diagram provides another way of looking at your overall nutrition. A food pyramid illustrates the types of food to eat and the consumption quantities of each type of food. The United States Department of Agriculture (USDA) has published two food pyramids over the last seventeen years, and The Healthy Eating Pyramid was published in 2008.[57]

The USDA's 1992 food guide is the most recognized food pyramid in the United States. This food pyramid is shown below so you can understand how many ideas about what we eat have changed. Each of these food pyramids illustrates the importance of a diet rich in fiber and low in saturated fat. While there is much known about the benefits of low amounts of saturated fat and high fiber, we are always learning more, because the study of our health is an ongoing process after all.

1992 USDA Food Pyramid:

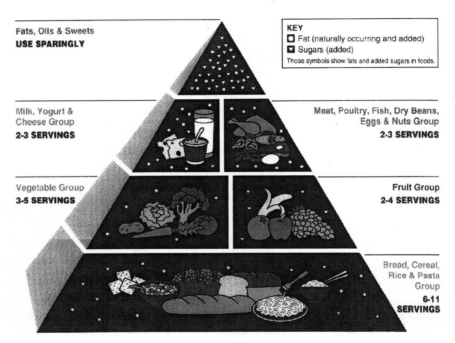

In April 2005 the USDA published a new food pyramid packed full of information. This food pyramid updated the 1992 version and included a stepping visual to signify the importance of exercise. The food information is divided into sections with guidance provided on each food group. This new pyramid is shown on the following page:

2005 USDA Food Pyramid:

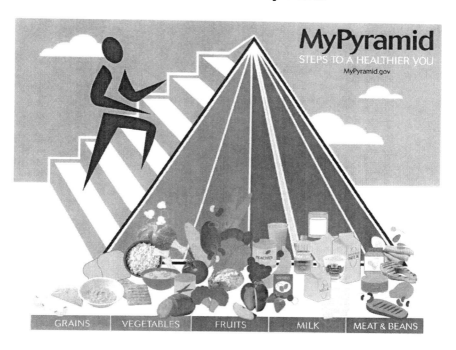

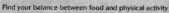

GRAINS Make half your grains whole	VEGETABLES Vary your veggies	FRUITS Focus on fruits	MILK Get your calcium-rich foods	MEAT & BEANS Go lean with protein
Eat at least 3 oz. of whole-grain cereals, breads, crackers, rice, or pasta every day 1 oz. is about 1 slice of bread, about 1 cup of breakfast cereal, or ½ cup of cooked rice, cereal, or pasta	Eat more dark-green veggies like broccoli, spinach, and other dark leafy greens Eat more orange vegetables like carrots and sweetpotatoes Eat more dry beans and peas like pinto beans, kidney beans, and lentils	Eat a variety of fruit Choose fresh, frozen, canned, or dried fruit Go easy on fruit juices	Go low-fat or fat-free when you choose milk, yogurt, and other milk products If you don't or can't consume milk, choose lactose-free products or other calcium sources such as fortified foods and beverages	Choose low-fat or lean meats and poultry Bake it, broil it, or grill it Vary your protein routine — choose more fish, beans, peas, nuts, and seeds

For a 2,000-calorie diet, you need the amounts below from each food group. To find the amounts that are right for you, go to MyPyramid.gov.

Eat 6 oz. every day	Eat 2 ½ cups every day	Eat 2 cups every day	Get 3 cups every day; for kids aged 2 to 8, it's 2	Eat 5½ oz. every day

Find your balance between food and physical activity
- Be sure to stay within your daily calorie needs.
- Be physically active for at least 30 minutes most days of the week.
- About 60 minutes a day of physical activity may be needed to prevent weight gain.
- For sustaining weight loss, at least 60 to 90 minutes a day of physical activity may be required.
- Children and teenagers should be physically active for 60 minutes every day, or most days.

Know the limits on fats, sugars, and salt (sodium)
- Make most of your fat sources from fish, nuts, and vegetable oils.
- Limit solid fats like butter, margarine, shortening, and lard, as well as foods that contain these.
- Check the Nutrition Facts label to keep saturated fats, trans fats, and sodium low.
- Choose food and beverages low in added sugars. Added sugars contribute calories with few, if any, nutrients.

MyPyramid.gov
STEPS TO A HEALTHIER YOU

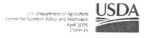

U.S. Department of Agriculture
Center for Nutrition Policy and Promotion
April 2005
CNPP-15

Finally, look at The Healthy Eating Pyramid, which gives a comprehensive health and wellness overview with a very good visual representation.

The Healthy Eating Pyramid

Department of Nutrition, Harvard School of Public Health

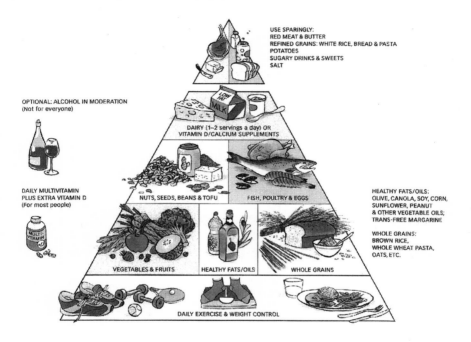

USE SPARINGLY:
RED MEAT & BUTTER
REFINED GRAINS: WHITE RICE, BREAD & PASTA
POTATOES
SUGARY DRINKS & SWEETS
SALT

OPTIONAL: ALCOHOL IN MODERATION
(Not for everyone)

DAILY MULTIVITAMIN
PLUS EXTRA VITAMIN D
(For most people)

DAIRY (1–2 servings a day) OR
VITAMIN D/CALCIUM SUPPLEMENTS

NUTS, SEEDS, BEANS & TOFU   FISH, POULTRY & EGGS

HEALTHY FATS/OILS:
OLIVE, CANOLA, SOY, CORN,
SUNFLOWER, PEANUT
& OTHER VEGETABLE OILS;
TRANS-FREE MARGARINE

WHOLE GRAINS:
BROWN RICE,
WHOLE WHEAT PASTA,
OATS, ETC.

VEGETABLES & FRUITS   HEALTHY FATS/OILS   WHOLE GRAINS

DAILY EXERCISE & WEIGHT CONTROL

For more information about the Healthy Eating Pyramid:

WWW.THE NUTRITION SOURCE.ORG

Eat, Drink, and Be Healthy
by Walter C. Willett, M.D. and Patrick J. Skerrett (2005)
Free Press/Simon & Schuster Inc.

Copyright © 2008 Harvard University

Copyright 2008. For more information about The Healthy Eating Pyramid, please see The Nutrition Source, Department of Nutrition, Harvard School of Public Health, http://www.thenutritionsource.org, and *Eat, Drink, and Be Healthy* by Walter C. Willett, MD, and Patrick J. Skerrett (2005), Free Press/Simon & Schuster, Inc.

There are several very important comparisons to make between The

Healthy Eating Pyramid and the first USDA illustration. Notice the shift in eating refined grains, white rice, bread, and pasta. In fact, they have a complete opposite location on the food pyramid. The USDA chart has these foods at the base of the pyramid, but The Healthy Eating Pyramid has these foods at the point of the pyramid. This is my point—processed foods should be eaten sparingly.

Now look at the fats and oils. Fats and oils are at the point of the USDA food pyramid, which means we should consume them sparingly, but The Healthy Eating Pyramid has healthy fats and oils at the base of the pyramid for food items. This is yet another complete reversal in food consumption recommendations.

Examine again The Healthy Eating Pyramid. What dominates the point of the pyramid? Besides refined grains, salt, and sweets, you will find red meat and butter, which should be consumed sparingly. According to The Healthy Eating Pyramid, dairy products also should be consumed in limited amounts, but the beneficial fats, placed at the base of the food pyramid, can be consumed more often. This is the formula for "targeting the 10" in *The 10-20-30 Life Wellness Plan*. Avoid foods high in saturated fat, and consume the good fats.

What dominates the base of the foods in The Healthy Eating Pyramid? Essentially, what foods do they recommend we eat the most? The answer is fruits, vegetables, and whole grains. This is the source of your fiber and why you want to "triumph over the 20" in *The 10-20-30 Life Wellness Plan*. By following the "10" and "20" parts of the plan, you reduce your saturated fat intake and increase your fiber consumption, and consequently, you will pattern your life to match The Healthy Eating Pyramid.

Finally and most importantly, look at what The Healthy Eating Pyramid shows at the base of the chart. This is the most important aspect of health. Because it is at the base of the pyramid, experts recommend this activity be done most often to ensure a life of wellness—*Daily Exercise!* Rightfully, the need for strenuous physical activity for at least thirty minutes a day is the topic of the final chapter in your life wellness plan—"Thrive on the 30" of *The 10-20-30 Life Wellness Plan*.

Let's keep it simple. Remember that fabulous fiber is good for you. Incorporating fiber into your diet will result in eating well and the consumption of nutritious foods. You must "triumph over the 20" and get twenty grams or more of fiber a day by eating grains, fruits, berries, beans, vegetables, oats, nuts, and almost any plant-based food. Animal foods do not contain fiber. Use what you now know about the benefits of fiber, and your body will react to the improved nutrition. Fiber is your Pac-Man at work, helping to reduce the effects of aging and keeping you healthy.

These first two steps in *The 10-20-30 Life Wellness Plan* provide the nutritional one-two punch to knock out the bad foods and incorporate the good foods into your eating habits. Understanding these two steps helps you adopt a healthy nutritional lifestyle and guides you in the proper food choices. Combined with step three—exercise—you will have a plan that'll help you achieve a life of healthy living and personal wellness.

"Successful people plan far more than the average person. There is an explanation. It works! If you want to succeed, plan for success"
—Anna Pavlova

Thrive on the "30"

"Champions aren't made in gyms. Champions are
made from something they have deep inside them; a
desire, a dream, a vision. They must have the skill and
the will. The will must be stronger than the skill."
—Muhammad Ali

The last step in *The 10-20-30 Life Wellness Plan* is all about exercise,
and it's the best part—exhilarating exercise. The quality of your life,
how you feel, how long you live, how well you live, how much energy
you have, the level of stress you endure, and your feeling of self-worth
can all be determined by your will to exercise.

We all know exercise is good for us. Understanding all the benefits
and the positive physiological impact of exercise on the body can
definitely help motivate you to incorporate exercise into your life.
You have the choice to make your life more vibrant, productive, and
enjoyable just by exercising thirty minutes a day. In this competition,
you can be your own champion. Become the champion of your life, for
it is the most important race to the finish that you will ever compete
in.

The body was designed to move, and understandably, you must be
active to live a healthy life. Think of all the things you must do in your
life. Attending school is a must. Maybe you have a family, and perhaps
you are active in the community. You likely have a job that fills up
most of the day. You have to eat to survive. You shower and brush your
teeth as part of a daily routine. All of these things are essentials in your
life. You must develop a mindset that physical activity (i.e., strenuous

exercise) is as important and as much a part of your life as everything else you do.

From now on, exercise should be a non-negotiable item that you must accept as a habit in your life.[58] This part of the wellness plan may very well be the hardest part for many people. To overcome your resistance to exercise, take it on slowly, and try doing the things in your life that keep you happy and active. Even as you take these small steps to become more active, you will feel the rewards almost immediately.

If exercise still does not appear on your radar, think of your life. Exercise might save your life and likely help you live longer—not to mention the fact that it will probably enhance the quality of those years added. If you do not routinely exercise, you must develop the exercise habit. We are talking about a major and difficult behavioral change for someone who does not exercise regularly.

Start by putting one foot in front of the other. It could all begin with a simple walk around the block or a stroll down a wooded path. Let each small success build to the next one. You can modify and add to your level of exercise over months, even years. Turn your sedentary life into an active one at your pace and by your own way. Remember, however, you must adopt this exercise habit so that it eventually becomes a lifestyle behavior. Change your habits. Change your behavior. And incorporate exhilarating exercise into your life today.

Improving wellness with more focus on exercise

Too many people are sedentary, even though the body is meant to be active. Rewards in life come from hard work. Similarly, the rewards for the body are also a result of hard work. Physical inactivity, especially among teens and adults, is a national health concern in the United States.

Becoming physically fit involves engaging in a range of exercises so that you can transition from sedentary to physically active. Total fitness involves a range of activities, including cardiorespiratory fitness (walking, jogging, biking, and swimming), muscular endurance (hiking, rowing, skating, and gymnastics), strength (weight training), and flexibility (stretching). Assessing your total fitness is not done just by looking at your activity level. Total fitness also involves measuring your body composition, calculated as a percentage of body fat or BMI.[59]

The lack of exercise and the lifestyle of being a "couch potato" run counter to our physiological structures, and these are contributing factors in many health problems. Numerous surveys indicate the average American spends twenty-eight hours a week watching television. Out of that four hours a day, you can cut out one television show and invest that time in your life wellness. Go exercise. A sedentary lifestyle leads not only to physical atrophy but also emotional and spiritual atrophy as well.[60]

Studies have repeatedly shown the negative impact of physical inactivity, which is undoubtedly hazardous to your health. As highlighted above, exercise is not something most people want to do. According to James Rippe, MD, only about 20 percent of the population in the United States is physically active enough to actually attain health benefits from their activity.[61]

Remember that over 65 percent of adults are overweight or obese. We are a nation full of inactive, overweight people who are inflicting unnecessary illnesses upon ourselves by choice. The CDC and The Drug War Facts Organization Web sites list many of the main causes of death in the United States as of 2006:

- Lightning: 48
- Water, air, and transport accidents: 1,915
- Homicide: 18,573
- Poisonings: 27,531
- Suicide: 33,300
- Automobile accidents: 45,316
- Flu and pneumonia: 56,326

Society now seems to accept these respective totals as part of our way of life. Efforts are made to reduce these fatalities, but there is no real alarm over the statistics. What would happen if numbers in any of these categories suddenly elevated to hundreds of thousands? How would the government's policies and procedures change? What would most citizens do? What changes would be made in our daily lives?

Well, there are other categories that far surpass the above totals and yet seem to be accepted as part of our way of life as well. Annual deaths related to tobacco use number 435,000. Approximately 365,000 deaths occur each year as a result of poor diet and physical inactivity. In his book *Real Age: Are You as Young as You Can Be?*, Michael Roizen, MD, estimates that three hundred thousand people die per year because of weight-related illness.[62]

These numbers are staggering. What is more startling is the fact that these are areas related to life choices. Your habits, your behaviors, your lifestyle, and the consequences of your choices are causing health-related deaths. Use this wellness plan. Take control of your body and your life. And live a life of wellness.

Benefits of exercise and the physiological impact on the body

"If exercise could be packaged into a pill, it would be the single most prescribed and beneficial medicine in the nation."
—Robert Butler, MD, Chairman of the Department of Geriatrics and Adult Development, Mount Sinai Medical Center

Committing yourself to a lifetime of exercise is not easy. You might wonder what will benefit you in this effort and if it's worth it. Consider the above statistics and the fact that 80 percent of people do not get the amount of exercise needed to benefit their health. Maybe seeing the health benefits of exercise will motivate you. If the list of benefits is not enough of a motivator, why not take an easy and very relaxing test then?

Most people who do little exercise have a resting heart rate of about seventy-five to eighty beats per minute. Individuals who are well conditioned may have a resting heart rate of fifty-five to sixty beats per minute. Superbly conditioned athletes may even have heart rates as low as thirty to forty-five beats per minute. Exercise impacts the heart muscle just like any other muscle and makes it more efficient. If you work your heart properly, it will work better for you and your future health.[63]

But how do you determine your resting heart rate? The best time to measure your resting heart rate is when you wake up in the morning. Before getting out of bed, take your pulse and count the number of beats you feel in one minute. Determine your average over a period of at least three days. Your resting heart rate is an excellent indicator of basic fitness and a strong predictor of cardiovascular health.

Information on resting heart rates is available on the American Heart Association Web site (www.americanheart.org). The table below provides general fitness categories for men and women based on your resting heart rate.

Resting Heart Rate (beats per minute)

Fitness Level	Men	Women
Athlete	49-56	54-60
Excellent	57-62	61-64
Good	63-66	65-69
Above Average	67-70	70-73
Average	71-75	74-78
Below Average	76-82	79-84
Poor	82 and over	85 and over

The list of benefits related to vigorous exercise is extensive and impressive, one backed by scientific research on exercise as it pertains to various health issues. If exercise could be taken like a pill, it would be widely prescribed. Examine the below list of ailments, and see if this "pill" is worth taking:[64]

- **Coronary and arterial aging**: People who exercise regularly have significantly less cardiovascular aging and a lower risk of heart attacks and strokes regardless of genetic background.
- **Immune system aging**: Physical activity reduces the rate at which your cells age, and you are less likely to develop cancers when you exercise regularly. Moreover, with activity, microscopic cancers that do exist are less likely to spread.
- **Colon cancer**: Physically active individuals have been shown to have much lower rates of colon cancer.

- **Breast cancer**: Women who exercise regularly are a third less likely to contract breast cancer than those who do not exercise regularly.
- **Prostate cancer**: Men who exercise consistently have lower rates of prostate cancer.
- **Arthritis**: Moderate to vigorous exercise in conjunction with strengthening exercise eliminates many of the arthritic symptoms and makes joints younger.
- **Weight management**: Exercising both aerobically and with strength-building activities increases the burning of calories and enhances metabolic rates.
- **Diabetes**: Exercise helps increase the body's sensitivity to insulin, which in turn lowers blood sugar levels and decreases insulin production. Active people—even if they have a genetic link to the disease—are much less likely to develop adult-onset (Type II) diabetes as a result of regular exercise.
- **Osteoporosis and loss of bone density**: Any resistance activity strengthens muscles and increases bone density.
- **Falls and broken bones**: Studies show that those who exercise are much less likely to fall or sustain fall-related injuries.
- **Sleep-related disorders**: Adults who exercise fall asleep more quickly and sleep better than their sedentary counterparts.
- **Depression and anxiety**: Exercise also has significant emotional benefits, and it can help ease depression, anxiety, and other psychological disorders.
- **Stress management**: Regular exercise decreases stress response, which means that you are more relaxed, feel better, and better prepared to cope with life's stressful events.
- **Long-term memory**: Exercise helps improve long-term memory and brain function as well. It helps prevent the arterial aging that can contribute to the early onset of Alzheimer's disease.
- **Tobacco use**: Increasing exercise levels often help people quit smoking. Regular exercise can diminish nicotine cravings.

**"You can set yourself up to be sick, or
you can choose to stay well."**
—Wayne Dyer

Listed in the beginning of this book are some of the problems we face because of inactivity and poor self-care. The benefits of exercise listed above should be a great motivator for you, because it clearly documents the positive impact on the body just from taking the "exercise pill." For some who feel healthy now, many of these benefits may not seem relevant; however, you must always remember how essential it is to develop the healthy habits and good behaviors that will allow you to integrate exercise into your lifestyle, because the future payoff will be tremendous.

Numerous other references and studies have further substantiated the above list of preventative measures. Exercise sends a positive signal to the body, setting in motion hundreds of chemical reactions each time you exert yourself and sweat. Muscles and joints are strengthened. The brain benefits from the positive chemistry, and you are more resistant to hypertension and high cholesterol.

It is well known that exercise reduces death from vascular disease, but science has now shown that exercise can reduce the mortality related to certain cancers as well. Cancer is an immune, inflammatory, and lifestyle disease related to decay. Exercise reverses the chemistry of decay and changes the blood. Do not let your muscles sit idle, because they will then no longer receive the positive growth signals so necessary for maintaining a healthy body. Choose fitness, for you then will become the recipient of its benefits.[65]

It can be hard to choose fitness, but good things come from hard work. Remember the quote by Matthew Kelly: "If you do only what you feel like doing, your life will be miserable, and you will be a failure." You must measure the benefits of exercise by how you feel *after* you exercise.

Think of how you feel before you become active for the day and how hard it can be to start exercising. But how do you feel after you exercise? Most people get a sense of personal satisfaction and feel physically better after they become active. The psychological benefits of exercise are often just as profound as the biological benefits. Physical activity helps clear the mind and burn off excess stress, and it also helps you feel good about yourself as a person.

"A vigorous five-mile walk will do more good for an unhappy but otherwise healthy adult than all the medicine and psychology in the world."
—Paul Dudley White

Naturally, you are going to feel better when you exercise. You may not notice it right away, but over time, you will value the elevated feelings associated with great workouts. As you challenge yourself, set new goals and achieve levels of fitness you never reached before. Your confidence will noticeably increase as well. These feelings transcend all ages, ranging from children to teens, from adults to the elderly.[66]

The psychological benefits of exercise definitely help students in school, too. Studies published in 2007 by the American College of Sports Medicine (ACSM) linked vigorous physical activity to better grades in school. Active students achieve more, become more focused, and show a psychological benefit resulting in improved academic performance. Michael Bracko, EdD, a fellow of the ACSM, shows that students who exercise are less likely to engage in negative social behaviors, such as smoking, substance abuse, premarital sex, or other misbehaviors that could negatively impact their life wellness.[67]

Maybe all these good feelings are tied to the actual changes taking place in the brain after you exercise. Physical activity—even walking—helps keep memories intact. Strength training and aerobics keep the mind sharp and increase the amount of gray matter (or more specifically neurons) in as little as six months. All these biological benefits help the brain plan, remember, and multitask better. It is logical to conclude that exercise has a positive impact on many aspects of individual performance. That said, these results need to be understood for the significance of what has been discovered—you can build new brain cells by exercising![68/69]

As if all these benefits are not enough—there's more! There is now information that strongly suggests that exercise lengthens life, which seems obvious as indicated by all of these physiological, biological, and psychological benefits.

A large scale study published in the *Journal of the American Medical Association* gave evidence that proved the age-adjusted death rate from all causes was nearly forty per ten thousand for women who got low amounts of exercise. In comparison, the death rate for women who got moderate daily exercise was less than five per ten thousand. These numbers indicate that no matter what the cause of death, the death rate is reduced by over 85 percent for those who exercise. This data supports the fact that the benefits of exercise do help extend life. These same trends that showed the benefits of exercise were found in the men's study as well.[70]

Another study on people with diabetes showed that walking at least two hours per week reduced the risk of premature death by 39 to 54 percent. A finding published in the *Journal of the American Medical Association* (2007) indicated fitness level (regardless of weight) was the single strongest predictor of mortality risk. People with the lowest level of fitness were four times more likely to die than those with the highest level of fitness. Again, the data indicates that you are putting yourself at a higher risk for life-threatening health problems by not exercising. The numbers are in your favor when you exercise, and the message is clear. Moderate exercise can make a dramatic difference in your life expectancy and the quality of the life you live.[71]

Of course, I really want to motivate you to exercise, and that is a key goal in the "Thrive on the 30" chapter. Understanding exactly how the body reacts to exercise can definitely help motivate you. You should understand the science of the body so you know what is happening inside you each time you exercise.

Exercise positively impacts the body down to the cellular level. Everything the body does in response to a reasonable exercise regimen is beneficial. The brain, the heart, the muscles, the circulatory system, the body's metabolism, and its cell production system all respond to exercise. Essentially, your exercise energizes the body.

As most already know, the heart is the pump in your body. When you exercise the pump works faster, delivering more nutrients and oxygen to all body parts, including the brain. Many people believe exercise just affects muscles; however, studies now show that exercise improves the functions of the brain, too. People with the fittest bodies have the fittest brains as well. In fact, there is a growing acceptance in science that exercise can actually make people smarter.

With regular exercise the brain's nerve cells branch out, join together, and communicate with each other in new ways. In addition, exercise stimulates production of many beneficial chemicals in the brain, fueling the brain's thought-processing activities. Many people are aware of the impact of endorphins and their positive emotional feedback after vigorous exercise, which is often referred to as "runner's high."

The National Academy of Sciences documented results that showed the impact of exercise on the human brain. After three months of workouts, subjects in the study appeared to sprout new neurons, and those with the greatest cardiovascular fitness grew the most nerve cells.[72]

This process of transforming stem cells into full-grown, functional nerve cells is an exciting finding for the scientific community. Scott Small, a Colombia University Medical Center neurologist stated, "In terms of trying to explain what it means, the field is just exploding." He later continued, "Wherever you have birth of new brain cells, you have the birth of new capillaries, and active adults have less inflammation in the brain."[72]

Mary Carmichael's article, "Stronger, Faster, Smarter," cites several top medical researchers. One of those, Arthur Kramer, a psychologist at the University of Illinois, commented on how exercise seems to restore parts of the brain to a healthier state when he said, "It's not just a matter of slowing down the aging process; it's a matter of reversing it." These top medical researchers now provide sound scientific evidence to show that if you let your body go, the brain will follow.[72]

> ## "Physical fitness is not only one of the most important keys to a healthy body; it is the basis of dynamic and creative intellectual activity."
> —John F. Kennedy

The impact of exercise on those under twenty is even more dramatic. Phil Tomporowski, a professor of exercise science at the University of Georgia, says, "Exercise probably has a more long-lasting effect on brains that are still developing." Exercise benefits the brain by improving brain functions that include skills related to math, logic, and reading.[72]

There is a growing trend to examine the need for lengthening physical education and focusing on brain-strengthening cardiovascular exercise. Humans thrive on physical activity, and without this activity, our brains are not doing what they are meant to do. Kids need this activity for their brain health and development. By establishing a love of sport early in life, kids are more likely to develop into active adults.[72]

Most people understand the heart benefits from exercise. Exercise immediately does one thing to the heart. Increase your activity levels, and the heart suddenly starts to beat faster. If you are a conditioned athlete, a healthy heart can smoothly accelerate from sixty or seventy beats per minute to over 180 beats per minute. This remarkable pump then sends massive amounts of blood to exercising cells and tissue. Astonishingly, the flow of blood can even jump from one gallon per minute pumped to eight gallons a minute.[73]

The conditioning of the heart from exercising also impacts the heart's beating patterns. A person who routinely undergoes vigorous aerobic workouts can condition the heart so that his resting heart rate is reduced. With demanding aerobic exercise, the amount of blood pumped by the heart increases, too. This strenuous workout strengthens the heart, enlarges the left ventricle, and improves the ability of the heart to contract.

A heart routinely worked becomes more powerful and efficient as a result. As your fitness improves, your heart gets stronger and can pump a greater volume of blood with each beat. Thus, during normal activity, less beats would be required to maintain a functional body with a stronger heart.

As the heart pumps faster, the bloodstream and circulatory system also benefit from exercise. Think of your blood as the water in a river and your blood vessels as the banks of the river. How would you like this river in your body to function? Now picture a stream of fresh, clean water rapidly flowing along. Then picture a stream clogged up with debris, causing stagnant water, decay, and deteriorating conditions. Although the analogy concerns different scales, there is a similar process involved in the body.

With an increase in circulation, blood vessels become more flexible, and the small capillary vessels making up the network throughout the cells of your body increases. The blood also acquires more HDL (high density lipoprotein), and the good cholesterol levels as well as the overall picture of cholesterol are improved. All these physiological impacts on the body help reduce the risk of developing atherosclerosis.[74]

When you exercise hard, you stress your body and its muscles. Your workout causes your energy reserves to drain, and you actually injure your muscles slightly. But the body is amazing. It recognizes this "injury" and builds it back. You are essentially tearing yourself down to build yourself back up stronger.

This type of injury is called *adaptive microtrauma*. This physiological process is critical to your growth and health. Remember that you are getting stronger by stressing your muscles. The body is building more tiny blood vessels inside your muscles. You are choosing to "thrive on the 30," and you are sending signals to your body, keys in overriding decay. But it all starts with exercise. You have to routinely exercise for your entire life because it's who you are.[75]

Maybe the smallest living part of your body will provide you the most motivation to exercise. Your understanding of the physiological processes occurring at the cellular level could influence your decision to become more active. Medically, it has been proven that exercise changes the cells throughout the body at the genetic level.[76]

We still do not know all the medical facts about the body's response to exercise, and of course, there is much more to learn about the details of how cells in the body respond to certain stimuli. Cells in the body go through a process of forming and being replaced. For example, muscle cells in the thigh are replaced every four months. New muscles are formed three times a year, and bones are renewed every couple years. You get brand new blood cells every three months, and you receive new platelets every ten days. Every day, your taste buds are replaced as well. You are an ongoing reconstruction project.[77]

Henry Lodge, MD, author of *Younger Next Year*, provides one of the best descriptions of the biological functions of the body and the need to maintain a high level of fitness. In fact, Dr. Lodge provides a very thought-provoking summary of how the body responds to exercise. Read this passage carefully, and whenever you feel like sitting on the couch instead of going out to exercise, read it again:

> Biologically there is no such thing as retirement, or even aging. There is only growth or decay. This is the new biology that has forever changed our thinking

about aging. It is all about growth and decay. Biologists now believe that most cells in your body are designed to fall apart after relatively short life spans, partly to let you adapt to new circumstances and partly because older cells tend to get cancer, making immortal cells not such a great idea.

The net result is that you are actively destroying large parts of your body all the time and on purpose! Think of it as throwing out truckloads of perfectly good body to make room for new growth. Your spleen's major job is to destroy your blood cells. You have armies of special cells whose only job is to dissolve your bones so other cells can build them up. Think of it like pruning in autumn to make room for growth in spring.

The trick of course is to grow more than you throw out and this is where exercise comes in. Muscles control the chemistry of growth. The nerve impulse to contract a muscle also sends a tiny signal to build it up. If enough growth signals are sent they overwhelm the signals to atrophy and your body turns on the machinery to build up the muscles, heart, capillaries, tendons, bones, joints, coordination and so on.[77]

Obviously, you should understand how critical exercise is to the proper functioning of the body. The above excerpt highlights how to keep the body from deteriorating. Let your body know that you want your cells to constantly rebuild a stronger and better you. Eat proper foods so that your cells have the fuel they need to rebuild. And above all else, be committed and engaged in living.

The fundamental building block supporting all these health benefits is exercise. You must exercise routinely for the rest of your life. The body was meant to move and to grow, not deteriorate. This is how the body is designed to function. What is really amazing is that so little time is needed to reap the benefits of exercise. If you invest thirty minutes to an hour in exercise a day, your body will physiologically respond in such a positive way.[78]

Recommended amounts of exercise and fitness assessment tools

"Fitness is a journey, not a destination. It must be continued for the rest of your life."
—Dr. Kenneth Cooper, aerobics expert and founder (1970) of the Cooper Institute, a preventive medicine research facility

This discussion on how exercise positively impacts the body brings us to the point of this section: how much should you exercise? Exercise is the best part of *The 10-20-30 Life Wellness Plan*. Set aside thirty minutes of exercise a day. Establish an exercise regimen as a habit, and this behavior change will become part of your routine for the rest of your life. If you think there is no time in your life for exercise, you must reprioritize and make exercise part of your lifestyle. You're the one who needs to make it happen!

Updated recommendations from the American Heart Association and the American College of Sports Medicine call for at least thirty minutes of moderate-intensity aerobic activity five days a week or twenty minutes of vigorous activity (like jogging) three days a week.

Strength training is a necessary component of the exercise regimen as well. Resistance exercises improve overall fitness, burn fat, help joints function better, and increase total muscle mass. Complete a strength training workout twice a week on nonconsecutive days. Your workout should involve all major muscle groups, focusing on the arms, legs and torso. Use weights with enough resistance to complete only eight to twelve repetitions. Make sure to complete a couple of sets of each exercise, too.[79]

Setting goals is obviously important, and your objectives can be centered on the amount of time you exercise or the amount of exercise you do. Clear guidance is available if you want to quantify the amount of recommended exercise. A recently completed government effort, headed by thirteen top fitness experts under the direction of the U.S. Department of Health and Human Services, defines exercise guidelines in the same way that the food pyramid defines healthy diets. The thorough results of this effort are documented and available on the U.S. Department of Health and Human Services Web site under the National Physical Activity Guidelines.

Both the Centers for Disease Control and Prevention and the American College of Sports Medicine recommend adults accumulate at least thirty minutes a day of moderate-intensity physical activity on most if not all days of the week. The National Physical Activity Guidelines also support a similar amount of exercise and state most health benefits occur with at least 150 minutes a week of moderate physical activity.

Dr. William Kraus, a Duke University cardiologist and professor of medicine, is one of thirteen fitness experts who developed this national policy on physical activity. The consensus on what is important for overall wellness focuses on movement, not the intensity of your exercise program. Based on the results in the National Physical Activity Guidelines, the most important parameter is how much exercise you do, not how hard you do it.[80]

In addition, Dr Kraus recommended that the average American should walk or jog nine to ten miles a week. The equivalent biking would be forty-five to fifty miles a week, and swimming would equal about two miles a week.[80] These distances can easily translate to the time recommendations cited above.

The National Physical Activity Guidelines were developed to promote physical activity and healthy diets in order to reduce the risk of chronic diseases. These results are designed to provide guidance on the types and amounts of physical activity with the goal of providing significant health benefits. If you focus on the amount of exercise time and "thrive on the 30," you may become more successful in setting goals for yourself and following this wellness plan as part of your lifestyle.

Keep in mind the total requirements of your exercise plan. You must also be sure to combine the aerobic part with the strength-building part. You will live longer by combining strength-building and stamina-building exercises. You should complete strength-building exercises, such as weight training, two to three times a week for at least ten minutes each time. Do stamina-building exercises that boost your heart rate and aerobic intake at least twenty to thirty minutes three to four times a week.

You should exercise vigorously enough to raise your heart rate to 70 percent of the maximum for your age. Your maximum heart rate can be determined by subtracting your calendar age from 220 beats per minute. There are a variety of heart monitors that you can wear to track the heart's performance during exercise, but one way to easily estimate the 70 percent level is to do your workout until you break a sweat. Sweating is a relatively reliable indication that you have reached 70 percent of your maximum heart rate and that you are completing a workout to improve stamina and benefit your health.[81]

A simple, easy-to-follow, strength-building routine recommended by the American College of Sports Medicine and the American Heart Association is included in Appendix C. Pick an exercise like biking, swimming, walking, or jogging for your aerobic workouts. Appendix D provides a very simple, gradual workout routine to build up your conditioning to a basic level of jogging for twenty to thirty minutes.[82] You could also choose to just keep walking and build on your pace and distance. Moreover, you can develop similar plans like those in Appendix D for biking or swimming.

"I run because it's my passion and not just a sport. Every time I walk out the door, I know why I'm going where I'm going, and I'm already focused on that special place where I find my peace and solitude."
—Sasha Azevedo

Fitness testing is important, because you always need to assess your fitness level. As a productive person, you should be well rounded. You should be a leader at work, pursue learning, remain active in the community, and be focused on personal fitness. You should prepare and put effort into many of these areas every day. Like the quote above, you should get to a point where fitness becomes a special place for you. It may not be running, but you should find some fitness passion to keep you motivated. Doing an activity you are passionate about will in turn improve your conditioning, performance, and wellness.

You already take tests to evaluate your performance level in so many areas of life. Your health, wellness, and fitness are even more important. How fit are you? At the start of your fitness journey (or as you continue a conditioning program), you may want to determine your fitness level. A thorough fitness test measures *aerobic ability, strength, flexibility,* and *body composition.* This type of comprehensive fitness test is similar to what Pamela Peeke, in her book *Fit to Live*, recommends.[83] The U.S. Air Force also uses these same criteria to evaluate fitness levels.[84]

Walking or running fitness tests measure your *aerobic ability*. Push-up testing is used to evaluate your *strength*. Sit-up testing is provided to assess *flexibility* and middle-body strength. The waist measurement provides another test for *body composition*, and the results can be used to supplement your Body Mass Index assessment covered in the chapter "On the Nature of Wellness." (All of these assessment tools for both men and women are in Appendix E.) Each chart is proportionally scaled to help you determine your level of fitness, conditioning, and health. (Also included in Appendix F is a personal fitness assessment log to track initial fitness parameters and monitor progress on your journey in a life of wellness.)

Included previously were many factual and expert exercise recommendations from top professionals in the field of fitness and wellness. Let's keep it simple, too. Remember that there is a common theme to what these various doctors recommend and the relationship to the "Thrive on the 30" chapter. Most days of the week, you should exercise thirty minutes a day. You should alternate days between aerobic (stamina-building) workouts and strength-training (resistance-building) exercises.

Your aerobic workouts should be intense enough that you develop a sweat for at least thirty minutes. Your weight-training exercises should be done on all the major muscle groups, using weights that exhaust you with eight to twelve repetitions in two to three sets. This resistance training must stress the muscle enough to cause a change. Remember that you are trying to build your muscles and cells stronger than they were before, which may help motivate you as well.

The basic knowledge included in the previous chapters now affords you the power to make the right choices concerning nutrition and exercise. With all three steps of this wellness plan in place, you now have a framework to develop goals and a total wellness plan, which leads us to the last chapter on you, "All about Your Body, Mind, Soul, and Spirit."

"Do not let what you cannot do interfere with what you can do."
—John Wooden

All about Your Body, Mind, Soul and Spirit

"And in the end, it's not the years in your life that count. It's the life in your years."
—Abraham Lincoln

You need to be a little selfish here. Think about you for a change. Think about your life now, your life ten years from now, your life fifty years from now. You want to have quality life in those years, don't you? What you do, the wellness choices you make, and the commitment you make to yourself will make a huge difference in how your future life is lived.

One of the most important benefits of following *The 10-20-30 Life Wellness Plan* is the energy level you will feel throughout your lifetime. Think of the energy of that rapidly flowing stream mentioned in the previous chapter and compare it to the energy level of the stagnant swamp. No one can control the amount of time we each have in a day, but we do have control over the energy we put into that day.

Reflect again on the power of three. You now have a *simple wellness plan* based on "Target the 10," "Triumph over the 20," and "Thrive on the 30." You now possess the information you need to make educated decisions about how you can adopt a diet low in saturated fat and high in fiber. You know the benefits you will reap from a combined nutrition and exercise program, and you know how to make changes in your life to realize those benefits. You must make a *commitment* to yourself, placing personal wellness as a top priority in your life. You are unique. You must make wise decisions. You must do things right and with extra effort. Finally, you must *set goals*.

Setting goals is a must for *The 10-20-30 Life Wellness Plan*. More importantly, setting goals is really a must for all activities in your life. For the moment, consider all of the things you do every day and then think how you can be a better person by setting goals.

Your goals might be related to a work project or a to-do list at home. One of your major goals could be to further your education or develop a key presentation. Maybe you have financial issues to resolve and want to either pay off a major debt or save for a special purchase. Goals might help you get through a book you want to read or prepare yourself for something you fear, yet is necessary.

Even if you make a simple list of things to do for the day or the week, those are goals, too. Get into a habit of setting goals for yourself. You will find that a nurtured goal-setting behavior will apply to many areas and cover every activity in life. The point is you can maximize your efforts, energize your day, best utilize your time, and accomplish far more by setting goals.

"Far better it is to dare mighty things, to win glorious triumphs, even checkered by failure, than to take rank with those poor spirits who neither enjoy much nor suffer much, because they live in the gray twilight that knows not victory nor defeat."
—Theodore Roosevelt

Goals and motivation to live a life of wellness

"Go confidently in the direction of your dreams. Live the life you have imagined."
—Henry David Thoreau

Goals do not have to be complicated. Keep your goal setting simple. A good goal must be well defined, attainable, and measurable. Every area of life can be maximized by setting goals. Goals can be long term or short term as well. So too, a long-term goal can even set up many short-term goals. Setting goals is important in life, and it is equally important in achieving improved health through this nutrition and exercise plan.

When I first started this wellness plan, I knew that I needed to set goals in each key area—nutrition and exercise. Initially, I had trouble understanding everything that I needed to do, but I eventually found a simple way to implement my goals so that I could follow the plan for the rest of my life. I applied basic nutrition to my fat and fiber intake and kept at my goal-setting exercise regimen. All in all, the wellness plan I present here helped me overcome the obstacles that were preventing me from lowering my cholesterol, which enabled me to improve my overall health and fitness.

That said, setting goals can be applied to each area of this wellness plan. Let's combine the information in "Target the 10" and the "Triumph over the 20" in order to demonstrate the application of doable goals.

- <u>Month 1</u>: I will familiarize myself with nutrition labels and focus on the amounts of saturated fat and fiber contained in the foods that I tend to eat.
- <u>Month 2</u>: I will list the foods that I eat containing low amounts of saturated fat and high amounts of fiber for one week of the month.
- <u>Month 3</u>: I will track my daily amounts of saturated fat and fiber eaten for at least two weeks of the month.
- <u>Month 4</u>: I will maintain a daily log of saturated fat and fiber eaten for the entire month.
- <u>Month 5</u>: I will have established this pattern of eating so that I can mentally track these amounts, know which foods are nutritious, and maintain these eating habits for the rest of my life.

These goals are only examples. You should set goals that work for your particular lifestyle. The last goal listed above is not as measurable as the others, but the whole purpose here is to get you to the point where you can control your food choices so that these food selections become simple and easy to track without extensive record keeping.

After four months of familiarizing yourself with nutritious foods, you will develop the "saturated-fat-and-fiber mentality." The end goal is to have you so knowledgeable that the nutrition part of this wellness plan becomes automatic. You should eventually become aware of foods containing too much saturated fat, and you should automatically start to "target the 10," bringing saturated fat consumption down to about ten grams consumed per day. Your habits and your behaviors should become established as well so that you can "triumph over the 20" by increasing your fiber to at least twenty grams consumed a day.

Exercise is the perfect activity for the goal-oriented person. The simple goal here is to exercise at least thirty minutes a day during most days of the week. Consider how exercising can bring you benefits that will last your entire lifetime. As with nutrition, we are trying to establish a life wellness plan, so your exercise goals must be lifetime goals, thus changing behaviors and establishing patterns of living to ensure a life of wellness.

For exercise, it is important to establish the long-term goal first. This can be done using daily, weekly, and monthly goals. The Sample Workout Goals table on the following page provides an example of many goals for jogging, walking, swimming, biking, and strength building. The weekly distances are taken from Dr. Kraus's work with the National Physical Activity Guidelines project. (See "Thrive on the 30.")

You should select goals that match your abilities and what you think you can do. Can you walk or jog two miles in a day? Can you bike five miles? Figure out what you can do in one workout. Your aerobics workout should be done three to four times a week. You must also do strength-building exercises at least twice a week, preferably not back to back. Allow a day off each week to rest. This day off can fall on a day when events are just overwhelming you and you cannot fit in an exercise workout.

Next examine your weekly totals and finally set a yearly goal by multiplying your weekly totals by fifty. This allows a couple weeks off within the year and a cushion in case you get sick or injured. By setting long-term goals, which help establish short-term goals, you will not let exercise slip off your daily routine very often.

How would you train for a hundred-mile bike ride? You would first set the long-term goal of completing a hundred-mile bike ride. Then you would train and slowly increase the mileage you can cover over a period of time. Each of these smaller, short-term goals sets you up for the major event. It is these daily goals, which are met in the months before the ride, that make you a winner. Each goal must stretch your limits but also remain attainable. After all, you would not start training for a hundred-mile bike ride by going out and biking seventy-five miles on the first day.

You need to evaluate your ability and set your goal so that you are forced to reach a little beyond what you think you can do. Repeatedly doing this prepares you to meet challenges in life and to be ready when an opportunity surfaces. Success in life is often the result of being prepared when opportunity comes your way. Think of the second-string athlete, the understudy actress, and the fill-in singer. Would any of these people be successful when called upon if they were not already prepared? And once called upon, you will experience success if you are prepared, and you may even find more opportunities as a result.

To summarize, you should select a single aerobic activity or figure out a combination of aerobic workouts that work for you. Your aerobic exercises should generate sweat for at least thirty minutes for four times a week. You should complete a rigorous strength-building workout at least twice a week. Allow yourself one day a week to relax and recover. Based on this process, your goals can be established in a similar way as shown in the table below.

Sample Workout Goals

Activity	Daily workout	Weekly goal (aerobics-daily times 4)	Monthly goal (yearly divided by 12)	Yearly goal (weekly times 50)
Jogging	2.5 miles	10 miles	42 miles	500 miles
Walking	2.5 miles	10 miles	42 miles	500 miles
Biking	12.5 miles	50 miles	209 miles	2500 miles
Swimming	.5 miles	2 miles	8.5 miles	100 miles
Strength-building/weights	30-45 minutes	Twice a week	8-9 workouts	100 workouts

There is a tremendous amount of flexibility within the application of this table. It must be adapted to match your own abilities and interests. Most people should be able to construct something similar to match at least one of the listed activities. The key is to determine what you can do and what is comfortable in a single workout. Then develop your weekly totals, multiply it by fifty, and set yourself a yearly goal. You can adjust and modify your daily, weekly, and monthly goals as events unfold, but you should always have your yearly goal in mind.

By definitively knowing your long-term goals, you will become more motivated to continue building on your weekly and monthly goals as well. You can certainly mix and match your goals, participating in several sports and setting goals in each one. The crucial idea is to establish your own fitness goals in a workable plan. (As mentioned earlier, I have maintained a goal-setting exercise regimen over a long period of time. I have provided my aerobic goals and workout results in Appendix G to act as an example of setting goals this way.)

When you complete a year, examine how hard it was and ask yourself if you need to modify your fitness goals for the next year. Because this is a lifelong effort, there is no hurry, and each year your fitness goals may increase only a little or even stay the same. It is doubtful you will ever make the next year's goal less, for a goal-oriented person should always reach out to do a little bit more than before.

If you want to combine your exercise goal with a goal to purchase something at the end of the year, you can always pay yourself for each workout you complete. You might give yourself a dollar for walking or jogging a mile or five dollars for swimming a mile. Whatever you decide, find your fitness passion, make a choice each day to include fitness, have fun, and turn your life into one of health and energy.

"In the long run, we shape our lives, and we shape ourselves. The process never ends until we die. And the choices we make are ultimately our responsibility."
—Eleanor Roosevelt

A sample daily routine comparing lifestyles

How do your daily nutrition and exercise choices measure up? In a single day, you may make twenty-five to fifty key choices that will inevitably impact your wellness. Let's follow the daily routine of two people to examine this issue. These people could be students in high school, younger children, college students, adults, or those who are retired. I will use the example of two busy adults for this comparison, and refer to them as "Busy Person A" and "Busy Person B." The choices we make are indeed our responsibility, as you will see here.

"Busy Person A" gets up and prepares for another day at work. Getting up and allowing an extra fifteen minutes for a quick breakfast provides just enough time to eat a good meal and then drive to work. "Busy Person A" decides to have a bowl of Frosted Mini-Wheats with skim milk, a cinnamon roll with icing, and orange juice.

"Busy Person B" had to grab a quick meal on the way to work and stopped at a fast food place. It had been a hectic morning, and there was no time to fix anything, so this person made a quick stop and ordered a fast food meal for breakfast. "Busy Person B" orders a specialty sandwich with bacon, egg, and cheese. "Busy Person B" decides to also order whole milk to drink.

Both of these people settle in for a morning of work and their daily routine. By lunchtime, they are ready to make some more choices.

"Busy Person A" had known there was little time in the morning to get ready for work, so he packed a lunch the night before. "Busy Person A" decided to make a turkey sandwich on wheat bread, some carrots, a baggie of baked potato chips, and three Fig Newtons for dessert. "Busy Person A" grabs the bag of lunch and buys a fruit drink in the lunchroom.

"Busy Person B," however, makes the dash to the lunchroom, gets in line, and decides to order a large cheeseburger, french fries, and a fruit drink.

Both finish lunch and feel full enough to make it through the rest of the afternoon. After a day of work, each person is ready to head home, but they both decide to have a quick snack first, because lunch had seemed to wear off during the last conference meeting of the day.

"Busy Person A" chose to get an apple, a blueberry muffin, and a soft drink. That would be enough to get by and still not make him too full for a quick workout before dinner. An hour after he gets home, "Busy Person A" decides to go for a forty-minute bike ride on a quiet back road lined with trees. It is a route he has taken before, and though "Busy Person A" often times the workout, he decides on just taking a good hard ride today, building up a sweat as he goes up and down the hills.

"Busy Person B" feels really hungry and decides to snack on a Hershey's chocolate bar, some Flamin' Hot Cheetos, and a soft drink. It has been a long and tiring day, so "Busy Person B" decides to take a short twenty-minute rest and then watch some television until dinner is ready.

Both have now finished a full day of work and filled the late afternoon with individual activities. It is almost 6:00 PM, and they are ready for dinner.

"Busy Person A" opts to stay home for dinner instead of going out with friends. He had already planned the dinner for tonight, anyway. He also wants to attend an evening social activity later. For dinner, he eats a tossed salad, grilled chicken with brown rice, a sweet potato, and skim milk.

After work, "Busy Person B" lines up a get-together with friends before an evening community meeting. They then go out for pizza. "Busy Person B" decides to order a salad, a few bread sticks, three slices of pepperoni pizza, and a diet Coke.

Both fit in some personal time, reading or visiting with friends, before they attend their evening activities. By the time the evening events are wrapped up, it's pretty late, but there's still time to get a quick snack.

"Busy Person A" goes home, pops some popcorn, munches on some almonds, and drinks a coke. "Busy Person B," however, stops at the Dairy Queen with friends and orders a chocolate chip Blizzard before he gets home.

At the end of a long day, they brush their teeth, crawl into bed, and sleep soundly while they are recharging their bodies for another day.

It should be obvious which person is choosing to live a better wellness lifestyle. However, let's take a closer look at the results of this day's decisions and see what we can learn. The table on the following page itemizes the food choices and compares the "target the 10," "triumph over the 20," and "thrive on the 30" for each person's routine day.

"Busy Person A" and "Busy Person B"— Their "10," "20," and "30" Day

Meals for Busy Person A	Busy Person A Saturated Fat (grams)	Busy Person A Fiber (grams)	Meals for Busy Person B	Busy Person B Saturated Fat (grams)	Busy Person B Fiber (grams)
Breakfast			**Breakfast**		
Kellogg's Frosted Mini Wheats (24 pieces)	0	6	Sonic Toaster Bacon, Egg and Cheese	11	2
Skim milk	trace	0	Whole milk	5	0
Pillsbury reduced fat cinnamon roll with icing	1	0			
orange juice	0	0			
Lunch			**Lunch**		
Boar's Head mesquite wood smoked breast of turkey – skinless	0	0	Large hamburger with cheese	15	0
Arnold Brannola Country Oat (2 slices)	0	6	French fries-medium	4	4
Green Giant baby fresh carrots (1.5 oz)	0	1	Fruit drink	0	0
Lays baked potato chips (15)	0	2			
Fig Newtons (3)	0	0			
Fruit drink	0	0			
After-work snack			**After-work snack**		
Medium apple	0	4	Hershey's milk chocolate bar (.6 oz)	4	0
Sara Lee blueberry muffin	2	Trace	Flamin' Hot Cheetos (1 oz)	2	0
Soft drink	0	0	Soft drink	0	0
Dinner			**Dinner**		
All American tossed salad	0	2	All American tossed salad	0	2
Fat free honey mustard	0	0	Italian dressing (2 tbsp)	2	0
Grilled chicken (Tyson-8oz)	3	0	Pizza with pepperoni and cheese (3 medium slices)	15	6
Brown rice (1 cup)	0	4	Breadsticks (3)	3	Trace
Sweet potato with skin	0	3	Diet coke	0	0
Benecol (1 tbsp)	1	0			
Skim milk	0	0			
Evening snack			**Evening snack**		
Orville Microwave Smart Pop-1 serving	.5	4	Dairy Queen Chocolate Chip Blizzard	13	1
Almonds (25 or 1oz)	1	3			
Coke	0	0			
BUSY PERSON A TOTALS	8.5	35	**BUSY PERSON B TOTALS**	74	15
BUSY PERSON A EXERCISE	40 minutes	biking	**BUSY PERSON B EXERCISE**	None	

This scenario was selected to show a realistic and representative comparison. Certainly, your day-to-day routine may not be this structured and could include both healthy and unhealthy foods. Obviously, there are thousands of combinations that could be used in comparing daily wellness choices. The point of this single example, however, is to show how each food choice in a day can accumulate and make a big difference in the nutrition totals at the end of a day.

Each wellness choice during the day is important. For "Busy Person A," his choices added up and fell on the good side of the table, with thirty-five grams of fiber and only 8.5 grams of saturated fat. For "Busy Person B," however, his choices totaled seventy-four grams of saturated fat, which may be typical of some people but is nevertheless extremely excessive and unhealthy. For that matter, the lack of fiber in his diet indicates poor nutrition choices as well.

"Busy Person A" has a habit of exercise and likely a routine that has resulted in accumulating exercise time day after day, month after month. This behavior energizes the body, builds healthy cells, and sends the body the signal for growth. A rest at the end of the day may feel good but gets you no physical activity. "Busy Person B" gets no exercise day after day, month after month, and he is sending the body the signal of deterioration.

This "daily routine" example demonstrates how the choices you make every day impact your wellness. You must get into the proper mindset to constantly assess what you are eating and how often you are exercising. By focusing on only two key nutrition factors, you can simplify the process. Obviously, by developing the "saturated-fat-and-fiber mentality," you are not tracking everything—sugar content, salt content, complex carbohydrates, and excessive calories are not monitored—but if you keep in mind the saturated fat and fiber consumption in your diet, you will automatically get rid of the bad foods in your diet and consequently consume the good foods.

It is difficult for most people to follow a complete wellness plan and virtually impossible to constantly track everything year after year. It is much easier, however, to keep the "10," "20," and "30" in mind, and applying this process will definitely improve your wellness, keep you eating properly, keep you focused on exercise, and likely cover about 80 percent of what you need to do to maintain a nutritious and healthy lifestyle.

"Busy Person A" was also able to fit in a vigorous, forty-minute bike ride into his hectic day. Naturally, exercise is the foundation of your entire wellness plan. It is even the base of The Healthy Eating Pyramid, and it is the fundamental component of your lifelong wellness. Make exercise your top priority, for it is as important as eating, breathing, and drinking water. You must be active. You must develop a high energy level. After all, it is what your body is meant to do.

What is it like to live a life focused on the body, mind, soul, and spirit? Maybe those who live to be a hundred years old know this better than anyone does. Researchers have found certain traits common in centenarians (listed in Appendix H)[85] that support this claim as well. Living a well-rounded life with a holistic lifestyle is part of the answer to the question of longevity. The three steps of this wellness plan are also key habits found in those who have lived long, full lives.

How do you apply *The 10-20-30 Life Wellness Plan* so that your life becomes the best one it can be? It is a body, mind, soul, and spirit process, a holistic approach. Each of these areas in life must routinely be challenged, stretched, and allowed to grow. Your body can do more than you think. Take control of your thoughts first. Set your goals in thought, envision success in areas you never imagined, and transfer those thoughts into actions. The mind directs the body, and you will feel the rewards of this wellness plan in your soul as it lifts your spirit and elevates and energizes your life.

Each of us is unique. Find the uniqueness in you. Find your own fitness passion, and let this plan become part of who you are. Use this easy nutrition and exercise plan to improve your life. Combine your special talents with discipline to generate success in the "10," "20," and "30" areas of wellness and to integrate the process into your life.

Let your mind imagine living a rich, vibrant, and healthy life. Embrace what you have read, and put this plan into action for your own well-being. With this three-step plan, you have the basic knowledge necessary to live a life of wellness and make good choices. Use this commonsense solution every day for the rest of your life, and make the best of the time you have on Earth.

"It's a funny thing about life; if you refuse to accept anything but the best, you very often get it."
—Somerset Maugham

Appendix A

Personal Health Statistics

**The Total Cholesterol Chart Shows a
Type of Fat Found in the Blood
(Under 200 Is Optimum)**

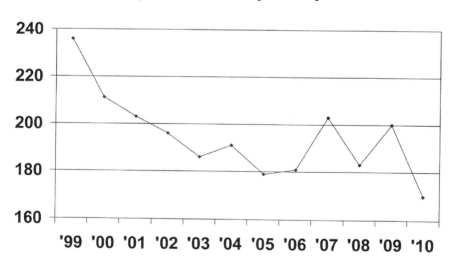

The Total Triglycerides Chart Shows
Another Type of Fat in the Blood
(Best If Totals Are under 150)

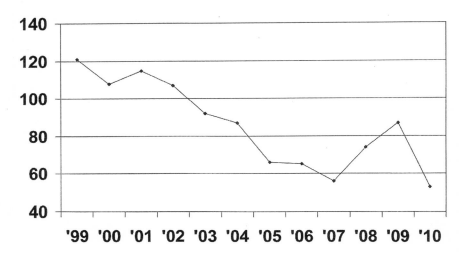

The HDL Chart Shows the Good Cholesterol Molecules
(Values over Forty Are Better)

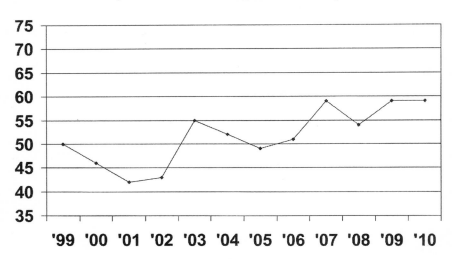

The LDL Chart Shows the Bad Cholesterol Molecules (Under a Hundred Is Best)

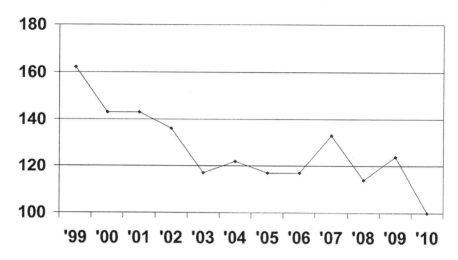

The Cholesterol/HDL Ratio Chart Represents Healthy Cholesterol Readings If the Ratio Is Less than Five

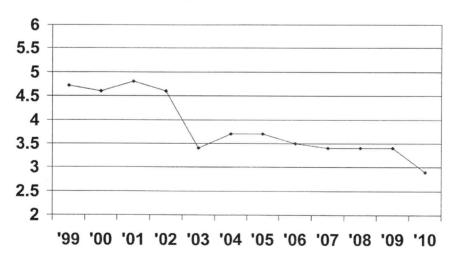

Appendix B

General Body Fat Percentage Categories

Classification	Women (% fat)	Men (% fat)
Essential fat	10-13%	2-5%
Athletes	14-20%	6-13%
Fitness	21-24%	14-17%
Acceptable	25-31%	18-25%
Obese	32% plus	25% plus

Appendix C

Recommended Strength Building Workout Routine

The American College of Sports Medicine (ACSM) and the American Heart Association (AHA) provide the following recommendations on strength workouts. These are the basics and provide a very simple way to get started. You can visit their Web sites at the following addresses: www.acsm.org and www.americanheart.org.

Terminology:

Rep is short for repetition, which refers to the amount of times you lift the weight.

Set means a group of repetitions.

Rest should be approximately one to two minutes between sets of each exercise (or long enough to catch your breath).

Muscle Groups to Target:

It is important to exercise the major muscle groups to develop your overall fitness.

- For the *upper body*, you should work the front and back of the arms, shoulders, and upper back.
- For the torso, you should work the *abdominals*, the sides of torso (obliques), and the lower back.
- For the *legs*, you should work the front and back of the thighs, the calves, and the buttocks.

Upper Body Exercises:

To keep the strength-building routine simple, use these five main *upper body* weight-lifting exercises to work the major muscle groups listed above.

Bicep Curls:

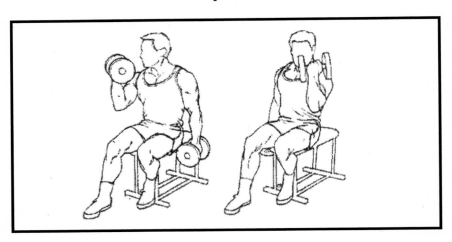

Shoulder Press:

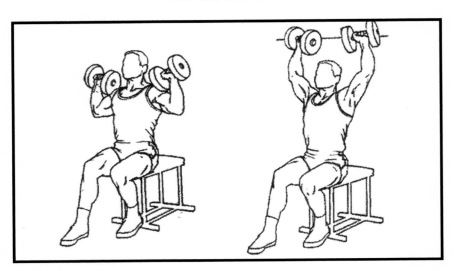

Tricep Extension:

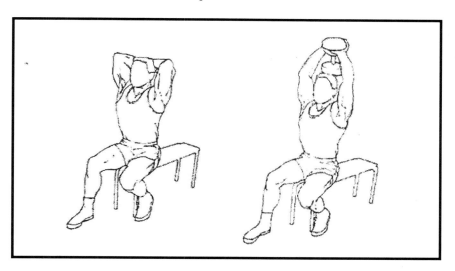

Bench Press:

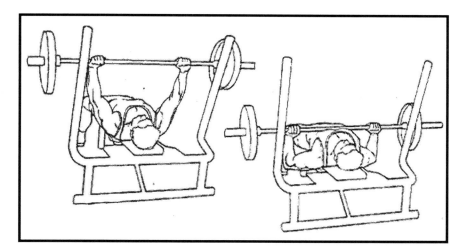

Bent-Over Row:

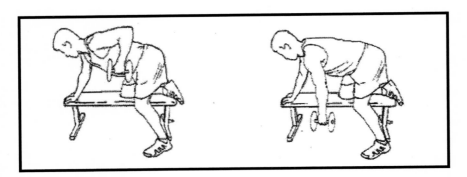

Abdominal Exercises:

For the torso, perform *abdominal* curls (with hands across chest or shoulders), side plank exercises, or the "Bird Dog," which is an exercise where you position yourself on your hands and knees and lift your opposite arm and leg with repeated reps.

Leg Exercises:

Perform squats or lunges to work major *leg* muscles

Lunge:

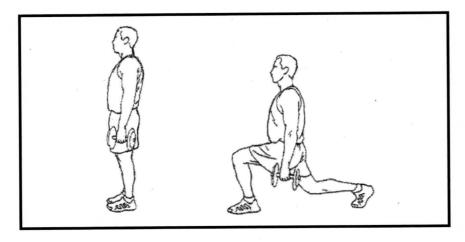

Technique:

Your strength-training workouts are as important for the joints as they are for the muscles. Be sure to follow the proper technique for each exercise, concentrating on form. Always exercise both sides of the body equally. Your breathing technique is also important. Exhale when the exercise is the most difficult, and inhale when you are performing the easier part of the exercise. Do not overexert yourself or perform a routine when your form is compromised. Exercise using your full range of motion so that your joints get a good workout, too.

Weight-Lifting Workout:

Weight-lifting workouts can improve muscle strength, endurance, or power depending on how you perform the reps and sets. These workouts are listed below:

- For muscle strength, perform five to eight reps with one to three sets.
- For muscle endurance, perform fifteen to twenty reps with one to three sets.
- For muscle power, perform three to five reps with one to three sets.

Remember the amount of weight to use must exhaust you and stress the muscles enough to cause change. You are working to grow and strengthen your muscles as well as your cells.

Appendix D

Recommended Aerobic-Building Workout Routine[82]

The following is a basic and simple routine to ease you into jogging as an exercise workout. After you have established your routine, you can then continue to add more time or miles to your workouts, or you can level off at about twenty to thirty minutes per session. Jogging is a very time-efficient way of getting a good aerobic workout at a level that benefits the body (a sweat-producing workout). Running puts a lot of stress on the lower body, so you should allow your bones, muscles, and joints to adapt as you go. Take the time to build up and strengthen your body. Remember that you want growth, not deterioration! Also remember that the body has the capacity to do more than you think, and after twenty-eight days, you may be able to make this fitness behavior a habit so that you can successfully implement a life of fitness and wellness. Remember to take it slowly. After all, you have lots of time.

	Mon	Tue	Wed	Thu	Fri	Sat	Sun
Week one	Walk 20 minutes	Off	Walk 20 minutes	Off	Walk 9 minutes, jog 2 minutes, walk 9 minutes	Off	Walk 8 minutes, jog 4 minutes, walk 8 minutes
Week two	Walk 25 minutes	Off	Walk 7 minutes, jog 6 minutes, walk 7 minutes	Off	Walk 4 minutes, jog 4 minutes, walk 4 minutes, jog 4 minutes, walk 4 minutes	Off	Walk 4 minutes, jog 5 minutes, walk 4 minutes, jog 5 minutes, walk 4 minutes
Week three	Walk 30 minutes	Off	Walk 6 minutes, jog 8 minutes, walk 6 minutes	Walk 20 minutes	Walk 3 minutes, jog 6 minutes, walk 3 minutes, jog 6 minutes, walk 3 minutes	Off	Walk 5 minutes, jog 10 minutes, walk 5 minutes
Week four	Off	Walk 2 minutes, jog 8 minutes, walk 2 minutes, jog 8 minutes, walk 2 minutes	Walk 30 minutes	Walk 4 minutes, jog 12 minutes, walk 4 minutes	Walk 4 minutes, jog 12 minutes, walk 4 minutes	Walk 30 minutes	Jog 20 minutes

Appendix E
Fitness Assessment Tools[83/84]

This appendix provides fitness assessment tools so that you can evaluate your *aerobic* ability (a one-mile walk or a 1.5-mile run), a basic *strength* test (regular push-ups for males and females), *flexibility* and core body strength (sit-ups), and another test for *body composition* (waist measurement), which can be used in combination with the BMI test discussed in the chapter titled "On the Nature of Wellness."

Aerobic Ability—One-Mile Walk Fitness Test
(Rating Based on Minutes by Age and Gender)

Rating	Men Under 40	Men Over 40	Women Under 40	Women Over 40
Excellent	13:00 or less	14:00 or less	13:30 or less	14:30 or less
Good	13:01-15:30	14:01-16:30	13:31-16:00	14:31-17:00
Average	15:31-18:00	16:31-19:00	16:01-18:30	17:01-19:30
Below Average	18:01-19:30	19:01-21:30	18:31-20:00	19:31-22:00
Low	Over 19:30	Over 21:30	Over 20:00	Over 22:00

Aerobic Ability—1.5-Mile Run for Women

Time is categorized by age group in minutes with rating and health risk. The health risk category is related to the risk for future cardiovascular disease, diabetes, certain cancers, and other health problems. The "*" placed in the table is the recommended passing level for this test.

Under 30	30-39	40-49	50-59	60 and over	Rating	Health risk
Less than 10:23	Less than 10:51	Less than 11:22	Less than 12:53	Less than 14:00	Superior	Low risk
10:24 to 10:51	10:52 to 11:22	11:23 to 11:56	12:54 to 13:36	14:01 to 14:52	Superior	Low risk
10:52 to 11:06	11:23 to 11:38	11:57 to 12:14	13:37 to 14:00	14:53 to 15:20	Superior	Low risk
11:07 to 11:22	11:39 to 11:56	12:15 to 12:33	14:01 to 14:25	15:21 to 15:50	Excellent	Low risk
11:23 to 11:38	11:57 to 12:14	12:34 to 12:53	14:26 to 14:52	15:51 to 16:22	Excellent	Low risk
11:39 to 11:56	12:15 to 12:33	12:54 to 13:14	14:53 to 15:20	16:23 to 16:57	Excellent	Low risk
11:57 to 12:14	12:34 to 12:53	13:15 to 13:36	15:21 to 15:50	16:58 to 17:34	Excellent	Low risk
12:15 to 12:33	12:54 to 13:14	13:37 to 14:00	15:51 to 16:22	17:35 to 18:14	Excellent	Low risk
12:34 to 12:53	13:15 to 13:36	14:01 to 14:25	16:23 to 16:57	18:15 to 18:30	Good	Low risk
12:54 to 13:14	13:37 to 14:00	14:26 to 14:52	16:58 to 17:14	18:31 to 18:56	Good	Low risk
13:15 to 13:36	14:01 to 14:25	14:53 to 15:20	17:15 to 17:34	18:57 to 19:15	Good	Low risk
13:37 to 14:00	14:26 to 14:52	15:21 to 15:50	17:35 to 18:14	19:16 to 19:43	Good	Low risk
14:01 to 14:25	14:53 to 15:20	15:51 to 16:22	18:15 to 18:33	19:44 to 20:33	Fair	Moderate risk
14:26 to 14:52	15:21 to 15:50	16:23 to 16:57	18:34 to 18:56	20:34 to 21:28	Fair	Moderate risk
14:53 to 15:20	15:51 to 16:22	16:58 to 17:34	18:57 to 19:43*	21:29 to 22:28*	Fair	Moderate risk
15:21 to 15:50	16:23 to 16:57*	17:35 to 18:14*	19:44 to 20:09	22:29 to 23:01	Fair	Moderate risk
15:51 to 16:22 *	16:58 to 17:34	18:15 to 18:56	20:10 to 20:33	23:02 to 23:34	Fair	Moderate risk
16:23 to 16:57	17:35 to 18:14	18:57 to 19:43	20:34 to 21:28	23:35 to 24:05	Poor	High risk
16:58 to 17:34	18:15 to 18:56	19:44 to 20:33	21:29 to 22:28	24:06 to 24:46	Poor	High risk
17:35 to 18:14	18:57 to 19:43	20:34 to 21:28	22:29 to 23:07	24:47 to 25:20	Poor	High risk
18:15 to 18:56	19:44 to 20:33	21:29 to 22:28	23:08 to 23:34	25:21 to 26:06	Very Poor	High risk
Over 18:56	Over 20:33	Over 22:28	Over 23:34	Over 26:06	Very Poor	High risk

Aerobic Ability—1.5-Mile Run for Men

Time is categorized by age group in minutes with rating and health risk. The health risk category is related to the risk for future cardiovascular disease, diabetes, certain cancers, and other health problems. The "*" placed in the table is the recommended passing level for this test.

Under 30	30-39	40-49	50-59	60 and over	Rating	Health risk
Less than 9:12	Less than 9:34	Less than 9:45	Less than 10:37	Less than 11:22	Superior	Low risk
9:13 to 9:34	9:35 to 9:58	9:46 to 10:10	10:38 to 11:06	11:23 to 11:56	Superior	Low risk
9:35 to 9:45	9:59 to 10:10	10:11 to 10:23	11:07 to 11:22	11:57 to 12:14	Superior	Low risk
9:46 to 9:58	10:11 to 10:23	10:24 to 10:37	11:23 to 11:38	12:15 to 12:33	Excellent	Low risk
9:59 to 10:10	10:24 to 10:37	10:38 to 10:51	11:39 to 11:56	12:34 to 12:53	Excellent	Low risk
10:11 to 10:23	10:38 to 10:51	10:52 to 11:06	11:57 to 12:14	12:54 to 13:14	Excellent	Low risk
10:24 to 10:37	10:52 to 11:06	11:07 to 11:22	12:15 to 12:33	13:15 to 13:36	Excellent	Low risk
10:38 to 10:51	11:07 to 11:22	11:23 to 11:38	12:34 to 12:53	13:37 to 14:00	Excellent	Low risk
10:52 to 11:06	11:23 to 11:38	11:39 to 11:56	12:54 to 13:14	14:01 to 14:25	Good	Low risk
11:07 to 11:22	11:39 to 11:56	11:57 to 12:14	13:15 to 13:36	14:26 to 14:52	Good	Low risk
11:23 to 11:38	11:57 to 12:14	12:15 to 12:33	13:37 to 14:00	14:53 to 15:20	Good	Low risk
11:39 to 11:56	12:15 to 12:33	12:34 to 12:53	14:01 to 14:25	15:21 to 15:50	Good	Low risk
11:57 to 12:14	12:34 to 12:53	12:54 to 13:14	14:26 to 14:52	15:51 to 16:22	Good	Low risk
12:15 to 12:33	12:54 to 13:14	13:15 to 13:36	14:53 to 15:20	16:23 to 16:57	Fair	Low risk
12:34 to 12:53	13:15 to 13:36	13:37 to 14:00	15:21 to 15:50	16:58 to 17:34	Fair	Moderate risk
12:54 to 13:14	13:37 to 14:00*	14:01 to 14:25	15:51 to 16:22*	17:35 to 18:14*	Fair	Moderate risk
13:15 to 13:36 *	14:01 to 14:25	14:26 to 14:52 *	16:23 to 16:57	18:15 to 18:56	Fair	Moderate risk
13:37 to 14:00	14:26 to 14:52	14:53 to 15:20	16:58 to 17:34	18:57 to 19:43	Poor	High risk
14:01 to 14:25	14:53 to 15:20	15:21 to 15:50	17:35 to 18:14	19:44 to 20:33	Poor	High risk
14:26 to 14:52	15:21 to 15:50	15:51 to 16:22	18:15 to 18:56	20:34 to 21:28	Poor	High risk
14:53 to 15:20	15:51 to 16:22	16:23 to 16:57	18:57 to 19:43	21:29 to 22:28	Very Poor	High risk
15:21 to 15:50	16:23 to 16:57	16:58 to 17:34	19:44 to 20:33	22:29 to 23:34	Very Poor	High risk
Over 15:50	Over 16:57	Over 17:34	Over 20:33	Over 23:34	Very Poor	High risk

Strength Test—Push-ups for Men

Begin in the up position with arms extended. The body must remain straight from head to heel. Lower the body to the level where the upper arms are parallel with the ground. One complete push-up is done upon the return to the up position. Rest may occur in the up position. Count the number of push-ups done in one minute. The "*" placed in the table is the recommended passing level for this test.

Under 30	30-39	40-49	50-59	60 and over	Rating
Over 67	Over 57	Over 44	Over 44	Over 30	Superior
66-62	56-52	43-40	43-39	29	Superior
61	51	39	38	28	Excellent
60	50	38	37	27	Excellent
59	49	37	36-35	26	Excellent
58	48	36	34-33	25	Excellent
57	47	35	32-31	24	Excellent
56-55	46	34	30	23	Excellent
54-53	45	33	29	22	Good
52-51	44	32	28-27	21	Good
50-49	43	31	26	20	Good
48-47	42	30	25	19	Good
46-45	41-40	29	24	18	Good
44-43	39-38	28	23	17	Fair
42-41	37-36	27	22	16	Fair
40-39	35-34	26	21-20	15	Fair
38-37	33-32	25-24	19-18	14*	Fair
36-35	31-30	23-22	17-16	13	Fair
34-33*	29-28*	21-20*	15*	12	Fair
32-31	27-26	19-18	14	11	Poor
30-29	25-24	17-16	13	10	Poor
28-27	23-22	15	12	9	Poor
26-25	21-20	14	11-10	8	Poor
24-23	19-18	13-12	9	7	Very Poor
22-21	17-16	11	8	6	Very Poor
20-19	15-14	10-9	7	5	Very Poor
18-17	13-12	8	6-5	4	Very Poor
Under 17	Under 12	Under 8	Under 5	Under 4	Very Poor

Strength Test—Push-ups for Women

Begin in the up position with arms extended. The body must remain straight from head to heel. Lower the body to the level where the upper arms are parallel with the ground. One complete push-up is done upon the return to the up position. Rest may occur in the up position. Count the number of push-ups done in one minute. The "*" placed in the table is the recommended passing level for this test.

Under 30	30-39	40-49	50-59	60 and over	Rating
Over 47	Over 46	Over 38	Over 35	Over 21	Superior
46-42	45-40	37-33	34-30	20-19	Superior
41-40	39-38	32	29	18	Excellent
39	37-36	31	28	18	Excellent
38	35-34	30	27	17	Excellent
37	33	29	26	17	Excellent
36	32	28	25	17	Excellent
35	31	27	24	16	Good
34	30-29	26-25	23-22	16	Good
33-32	28-27	24-23	21-20	15	Good
31-30	26-25	22-21	19-18	15	Good
29	24	20-19	17	14	Good
28	23	18	16	14	Good
27	22	17	15	13	Fair
26	21-20	16	14	12	Fair
25	19-18	15	13	11	Fair
24-23	17	14	12	10	Fair
22-21	16	13	11	9	Fair
20-19	15	12	10	8	Fair
18*	14*	11*	9*	7*	Fair
17-16	13-12	10-9	8-7	6	Poor
15-14	11-10	8	6	5	Poor
13-12	9-8	7	5	4	Poor
11-10	7	6-5	4	3	Very Poor
9-8	6	4	3	2	Very Poor
Under 8	Under 6	Under 4	Under 3	1	Very Poor

Note: women may want to begin conditioning for this test using the bent leg push-up position and building on that until comfortable doing straight leg push-ups.

Flexibility and Middle-Body Strength Test—
Sit-ups for Women

Begin with legs bent at a 90 degree angle with your body and feet resting on the floor. Arms should be crossed over the chest with hands on the chest or shoulders. Feet should be held or secured in an anchored hold. Raise upper torso until elbows touch knees or thighs. One complete sit-up is done when torso is lowered and shoulder blades touch the floor. Hands must stay in contact with the shoulders or the upper chest at all times. Rest may occur in up position. Count the number of sit-ups done in one minute. The "*" placed in the table is the recommended passing level for this test.

Under 30	30-39	40-49	50-59	60 and over	Rating
Over 54	Over 45	Over 41	Over 32	Over 31	Superior
53-51	44-42	40-38	31-30	30-28	Superior
50	41	37	29	27	Excellent
49	40	36	28	26	Excellent
48	39	35	28	25	Excellent
47	39	34	27	24	Excellent
46	38	33	26	23	Good
45	37	32	25	22	Good
44	36	31	25	21-20	Good
44	35	30	24	19-18	Good
44	34	29	24	17	Good
43	33	28	23	16	Fair
42	32	27	22	15-14	Fair
41	31	26	21	13	Fair
40-39	30	25	20*	12*	Fair
38*	29*	24*	19	11	Fair
37	28	23	18	10	Fair
36-35	27	22	17	9	Fair
34	26	21	16	8	Poor
33	25	20	15	7	Poor
32	24	19	14	6	Poor
31	23	18	13	5	Poor
30	22	17	12	5	Poor
29-28	21-20	16-15	11-10	4	Very Poor
27-26	19-18	14-13	9-8	4	Very Poor
25-24	17-16	12-11	7	3	Very Poor
23	15	10	6	2	Very Poor
Under 23	Under 15	Under 10	Under 6	Under 2	Very Poor

Flexibility and Middle-Body Strength Test— Sit-ups for Men

Begin with legs bent at a 90 degree angle with your body and feet resting on the floor. Arms should be crossed over the chest with hands on the chest or shoulders. Feet should be held or secured in an anchored hold. Raise upper torso until elbows touch knees or thighs. One complete sit-up is done when torso is lowered and shoulder blades touch the floor. Hands must stay in contact with the shoulders or the upper chest at all times. Rest may occur in up position. Count the number of sit-ups done in one minute. The "*" placed in the table is the recommended passing level for this test.

Under 30	30-39	40-49	50-59	60 and over	Rating
Over 58	Over 54	Over 50	Over 46	Over 42	Superior
57-55	53-52	49-47	45-43	41-39	Superior
54	51	46	42	38	Excellent
53	50	45	41	37	Excellent
52	49	44	40	36	Excellent
51	48	43	39	35	Excellent
50	47	42	38	34	Good
49	46	41	37	33	Good
48	45	40	36	32	Good
47	44	39	35	31	Good
46	43	38	34	30	Good
45	42	37	33	29	Fair
44	41	36	32	28	Fair
43	40	35	31	27-26	Fair
42*	39*	34*	30	25-24	Fair
41	38	33	29	23-22*	Fair
40	37	32	28*	21	Fair
39	36	31	27	20	Fair
38	35	30	26	19	Poor
37	34	29	25	18	Poor
36	33	28	24	17	Poor
35	32	27	23	16	Poor
34	31	26	22	15	Poor
33	30	25	21	14	Very Poor
32	29	24	20-19	13-12	Very Poor
31	28	23	18-17	11	Very Poor
30	27	22	16-15	10	Very Poor
Under 30	Under 27	Under 22	Under 15	Under 10	Very Poor

Body Composition Test—
Waist Measurement for Men and Women

To measure abdominal circumference, locate the hip bone and the top of the right iliac crest. Place measuring tape horizontally around the abdomen. Ensure the tape is snug and parallel with floor. The measurement should be made at the end of a normal expiration. Abdominal circumference is measured in inches. Health risk category is related to the risk of future cardiovascular disease, diabetes, certain cancers, and other health problems. The "*" placed in the table is the recommended passing level for this test.

Men	Women	Health Risk Category
Less than 32.5	Less than 29.0	Low risk
33.0	29.5	Low risk
33.5	30.0	Low risk
34.0	30.5	Low risk
34.5	31.0	Low risk
35.0	31.5	Low risk
35.5	32.0	Moderate risk
36.0	32.5	Moderate risk
36.5	33.0	Moderate risk
37.0	33.5	Moderate risk
37.5	34.0	Moderate risk
38.0	34.5	Moderate risk
38.5	35.0	Moderate risk
39.0*	35.5*	Moderate risk
39.5	36.0	High risk
40.0	36.5	High risk
40.5	37.0	High risk
41.0	37.5	High risk
41.5	38.0	High risk
42.0	38.5	High risk
42.5	39.0	High risk
43.0	39.5	High risk
Over 43.0	Over 39.5	High risk

A test often used in conjunction with the waist measurement test for body composition is the waist-to-hip ratio. This test may also be an indicator for the risk of coronary artery disease associated with obesity. Measure the waist as described above. Then measure the hip girth.

Next, take the waist measurement and divide it by the hip girth. Ratio values of 0.9 or less for males or 0.8 or less for females are good to excellent. Ratios of 0.9 to 0.95 for men and 0.8 to 0.85 for women are average. Ratios over 1.0 for men and over 0.9 for women would be considered an extreme risk.

Note: You can visit http://www.topendsports.com/testing/tests/WHR. htm for more details concerning the waist-to-hip ratio.

Appendix F

Personal Fitness Assessment Log

Total fitness can be thoroughly measured with tests to assess *body composition, aerobic ability, strength,* and *flexibility.* The following log is provided so that you can document your initial status and personal progress as you continue your journey with life wellness. Enter the date, log your results, and track your progress.

	Date	Date	Date	Date	Date	Date	Date
Body Composition							
BMI Value (range of about 18 to 30)							
BMI Health Risk							
Waist Measurement (in inches)							
Waist Health Risk							
Waist-to-Hip Ratio (about 0.8 to 1.0)							
Waist-to-Hip Ratio Health Risk							
Aerobic Ability							
One-Mile Walk (time in minutes)							
One-Mile Walk Rating							
1.5-Mile Run (time in minutes)							
1.5-Mile Run Rating/ Health Risk							
Strength							
Push-ups (number in one minute)							
Push-ups Rating							
Flexibility							
Sit-ups (number in one minute)							
Sit-ups Rating							

Appendix G

An Example of Personal Fitness Goals

In 1991, I set a personal goal to complete a two-mile run at the age of ninety. That said, my current goal is to run many miles so that I will be able to handle two miles at ninety, because there will be a natural decline in my abilities with age. This is just one example of a goal that can keep you engaged in life. The chart below is my aerobic progress to date:

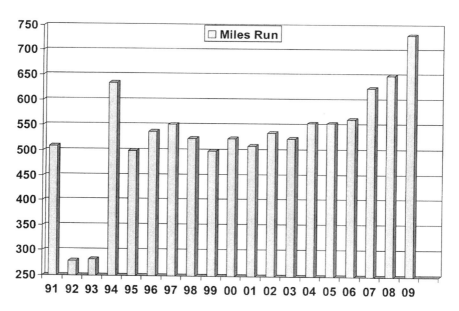

Since 1994, my goal for each year has been to run five hundred miles a year. Most years also included over a hundred weight-lifting sessions. This kind of achievement brings a great deal of personal satisfaction to me, and this dedication is a trait that I want to develop in each of you.

In life, it is important for everyone to set goals. Once you have a goal and achieve it, the internal satisfaction is self-rewarding and provides the drive and incentive to accomplish even more.

Make your goal attainable. Once met, your personal drive will ratchet the goal up a notch the next time. You have a long life ahead of you, and being successful with many small goals will eventually add up to a significant life achievement. Whether you focus on personal health, a business venture, or any life challenge, set a broad, overarching goal and then break it down into small, doable steps so that you can be successful in your endeavor. With life wellness, you can challenge yourself in many ways. Set goals, and realize a better future!

Appendix H

The Body, Mind, Soul, and Spirit Recipe for Longevity[85]

1. <u>**The Soul and Spirit**</u>: **Always be involved.** Even after you retire, stay busy. Studies show that the risks of obesity and chronic disease increase when people stop working. Stay active, volunteer, and get involved with people and activities. Energize your spirit, and keep your passion for life alive.
2. <u>**The Body**</u>: **Keep your gums clean.** Your mouth is a haven for bacteria. Research has linked high levels of bacteria in the mouth to problems with inflammation in the arteries and associated heart disease. If you floss your teeth each day, you can reduce the risks of gum disease and the bacteria related to poor mouth hygiene.
3. <u>**The Body and Mind**</u>: **Stay active.** The genuine fountain of youth is exercise. Every study done documents the tremendous benefits of exercise. Exercise positively impacts your muscles, bones, joints, sense of balance, and mental acuity. Even your mood and attitude will benefit. With only thirty minutes of exercise a day, you can change your life for the better. For aerobics, you can walk, jog, bike, swim, play tennis, or find any heart-healthy exercise. Do strength-building exercises with weights. Even yoga can have a strength-building effect on the body. Whatever path you take, you must always stay active.
4. <u>**The Body**</u>: **Eat fiber-rich foods.** Start your day with a high-fiber breakfast. A morning dose of fiber keeps blood sugar levels stable and lowers your likelihood of contracting diabetes. Fiber keeps the body young and helps maintain good health overall. Focus on whole grains and avoid highly processed foods.
5. <u>**The Body and Soul**</u>: **Do not skimp on sleep.** Sleep is the body's

way of recharging, healing, growing new cells, and regulating our internal rhythms. Getting to the phase of sleep that is needed for this healing requires about six hours. Don't overextend your day and miss sleep. Get more sleep to add years to your life.

6.   **The Body: Eat nutritional whole foods.** Nutrients in the blood—selenium, beta-carotene, and vitamins C and E—are linked to longer life and a slower rate of cognitive decline. The best way to get these nutrients is by eating fruits, vegetables, dark whole-grain breads, and whole-grain cereals. Taking pills with nutrients in them, however, is not as beneficial, and you should remember to avoid foods lacking nutrients like white foods (e.g., breads, flour, and sugar). Go for color in your foods, and get those nutrients the natural way.

7.   **The Mind, Soul, and Spirit: Live a less neurotic life.** Most people who have lived long lives have been able to better let go of their troubles, avoid internalizing problems, and "roll with the punches." Find ways to ease the mind as well as the soul and lift the spirit. When stressed, find some relief. Your uniqueness will determine your way of life. Relief may come from exercise, or it may come from yoga, meditation, quiet time, or just deep breathing. Feeling bad about yourself or your situation and eating junk food in front of the television will not help. Avoid bad habits as your cure, and find healthy ways to manage your stress.

8.   **The Soul and Spirit: Live a wholesome life.** Those of one particular faith, the Seventh Day Adventist, have an average life span of eighty-nine years, which is about ten years longer than the average American. They cherish the body as a gift and treat it with respect. They live a rich and well-rounded life, do not smoke or drink, and limit sweets. Their vegetarian diet is based on fruits, vegetables, beans, and nuts. They also get plenty of exercise and focus on family and community. Live a wholesome and spiritual life that enriches the soul, and the body and mind will also benefit.

9.   **The Body and Spirit: Live a life of discipline.** Develop good habits and stick with your good routines. Those with the most discipline in life are actually the happiest. Healthy routines of diet, exercise, and activities are important. Good sleep habits keep the body in

balance. Maintaining these habits keeps your immune system strong and makes you less susceptible to bacterial infections.

10. **The Mind, Soul, and Spirit: Keep connected to others.** Regular social contact with friends and loved ones is important in maintaining a healthy lifestyle and avoiding depression. Be involved, live life with others around you, and have daily connections with close friends or family members. Your role in their lives and their role in your life provides support, and this can help you stay focused on health and wellness.

Endnotes

1. Brian Wansink, PhD, *Mindless Eating* (New York: Bantam Dell, 2006), 213–217.
2. Howard Eisenson, MD, and Martin Binks, PhD, *The Duke Diet* (New York: Ballantine Books, 20070, 190–191.
3. Jordan Rubin, *Perfect Weight* (Lake Mary: Siloam, 2008), 15–21.
4. Study authored by Eric Finkelstein with RTI International an organization in Research Triangle Park, N.C. Results of study concluded that the greater the weight, the higher the medical costs. Published in *USA Today*, June 10, 2008, by Nanci Hellmich.
5. Pamela Peeke, MD, *Fit to Live* (New York: Rodale Inc., 2007), forward by former Arkansas Governor Mike Huckabee, vii.
6. Robert K. Cooper, *Low-Fat Living* (Emmaus: Rodale Press, Inc. 1996), 23–24.
7. Center for Disease Control and Prevention, results published in Associated Press article by Lindsey Tanner, May 28, 2008.
8. The American Heart Association, *A Nation at Risk: Obesity in the United States: A Statistical Sourcebook* (The Robert Wood Johnson Foundation, May 2005).
9. Pamela Peeke, MD, *Fit to Live* (New York: Rodale, Inc., 2007), pg. 4.
10. James M. Rippe, MD, *The Healthy Heart for Dummies* (Foster City: IDG Books Worldwide, 2000), pg. 32.
11. U.S. Department of Health and Human Services, Centers for Disease Control and Prevention, National Center for Health Statistics.
12. Michael F. Roizen, MD, *The Real Age Makeover* (New York: HarperCollins, 2005), pg. 242.
13. Chris Crowley and Henry Lodge, MD, *Younger Next Year* (New York: Workman Publishing, 2007), 31–32.

14. Michael F. Roizen, MD, *The Real Age Makeover* (New York: HarperCollins, 2005), pg. 239 and pg. 247.
15. Rick Galloop, *Living the Glycemic Index Diet* (New York: Workman Publishing, 2004), pg. 4.
16. Journal Report, American Heart Association, December 6, 2007.
17. Chris Crowley and Henry Lodge, MD, *Younger Next Year* (New York: Workman Publishing, 2007), pg. 14.
18. Chris Crowley and Henry Lodge, MD, *Younger Next Year* (New York: Workman Publishing, 2007), pg. 30.
19. Study done by the University of Cambridge in studying twenty thousand people in the United Kingdom, January 8, 2008. Published in the *Public Library of Science Medicine Journal*.
20. Brian Wansink, PhD, *Mindless Eating* (New York: Bantam Dell, 2006), pg. 214.
21. Gordon Livingston, MD, *Too Soon Old, Too Late Smart* (Philadelphia: Da Capo Press, 2008), 80–81.
22. John Izzo, PhD, *The Five Secrets You Must Discover before You Die* (San Francisco: Berrett-Koehler Publishers, Inc., 2008), pg. 116.
23. Mike Huckabee, *Quit Digging Your Grave with a Knife and Fork* (New York: Center Street—Time Warner Book Group, 2005), pg. 12 and pg. 41.
24. Chris Crowley and Henry Lodge, MD, *Younger Next Year* (New York: Workman Publishing, 2007), pg. 197.
25. Robert K. Cooper, *Low-Fat Living* (Emmaus: Rodale Press, Inc. 1996), 24–25.
26. Chris Crowley and Henry Lodge, MD, *Younger Next Year* (New York: Workman Publishing, 2007), pg. 14.
27. Pamela Peeke, MD, *Fit to Live* (New York: Rodale Inc., 2007), pg. 130.
28. Dorothy F. West, *Nutrition, Food, and Fitness* (Tinley Park: The Goodheart-Willcox Company, Inc, 2006), 221–222.
29. David Zinczenko, *The Abs Diet: Eat Right Every Time Guide* (New York: Rodale Inc., 2005), pg. 200.
30. Matthew Kelly, *The Rhythm of Life* (New York: Simon and Schuster, Inc., 2004), 176–178.
31. Bill Bryson, *A Short History of Nearly Everything* (New York: Broadway Books, Random House, Inc., 2003), 27–28.

32. Matthew Kelly, *The Rhythm of Life* (New York: Simon and Schuster, Inc., 2004), pg. 51.

33. Mike Huckabee, *Quit Digging Your Grave with a Knife and Fork* (New York: Center Street—Time Warner Book Group, 2005), pg. 140.

34. Air Force Junior ROTC, *Leadership Education I: Citizenship, Character, and Air Force Tradition* (Boston: McGraw Hill, Custom Publishing, 2005), pg. 207.

35. Annette Natow, PhD, and Jo-Ann Heslin, MA, RD, *The Most Complete Food Counter* (New York: Pocket Books, 2006), pg. 4.

36. David Zinczenko, *The Abs Diet, Eat Right Every Time Guide* (New York: Rodale Inc., 2005), 25–26.

37. Howard Eisenson, MD, and Martin Binks, PhD, *The Duke Diet* (New York: Ballantine Books, 2007), 37–41.

38. Chris Crowley and Henry Lodge, MD, *Younger Next Year* (New York: Workman Publishing, 2007), pg. 219.

39. Rick Galloop, *Living the Glycemic Index Diet* (New York: Workman Publishing, 2004), pg. 3 and pg. 77.

40. Michael F. Roizen, MD, *The Real Age Makeover* (New York: HarperCollins, 2005), pg. 69.

41. Gabe Mirkin, MD, and Barry Fox, PhD, *20/30 Fat & Fiber Diet Plan* (New York: The Stonesong Press, Inc., and LINX Corp., 2000), pg. 33.

42. Michael F. Roizen, MD, *The Real Age Makeover* (New York: HarperCollins, 2005, pg. 265.

43. Robert K. Cooper, *Low-Fat Living* (Emmaus: Rodale Press, Inc., 1996), pg. 37.

44. Dorothy F. West, *Nutrition, Food, and Fitness* (Tinley Park: The Goodheart-Willcox Company, Inc., 2006), pg. 101.

45. Chris Crowley and Henry Lodge, MD, *Younger Next Year* (New York: Workman Publishing, 2007), 222–225.

46. The National Fiber Council Web site: www.nationalfibercouncil.org

47. Howard Eisenson, MD, and Martin Binks, PhD, *The Duke Diet* (New York: Ballantine Books, 2007), pg. 24.

48. Annette Natow, PhD, and Jo-Ann Heslin, MA, RD, *The Most Complete Food Counter* (New York: Pocket Books, 2006), pg. 8.

49. David Zinczenko, *The Abs Diet: Eat Right Every Time Guide* (New York: Rodale Inc., 2005), 26–27.

50. Frances Sizer-Webb, Eleanor Noss Whitney, and Linda Kelly DeBruyne, *Health: Making Life Choices* (Chicago: National Textbook Company, 2000), pg. 175.

51. Dorothy F. West, *Nutrition, Food, and Fitness* (Tinley Park: The Goodheart-Willcox Company, Inc, 2006), pg. 103.

52. Rick Galloop, *Living the Glycemic Index Diet* (New York: Workman Publishing, 2004), pg. 6.

53. Gabe Mirkin, MD, and Barry Fox, PhD, *20/30 Fat & Fiber Diet Plan* (New York: The Stonesong Press, Inc., and LINX Corp., 2000), pg. 5 and 17–29.

54. Robert K. Cooper, *Low-Fat Living* (Emmaus: Rodale Press, Inc., 1996), pg. 45.

55. Michael F. Roizen, MD, *The Real Age Makeover* (New York: HarperCollins, 2005, 272–273.

56. ConsumerReportsHealth.org experts, "10 Tips for a Healthy Heart," *Consumer Reports* (May 2008): 40.

57. Chris Crowley and Henry Lodge, MD, *Younger Next Year* (New York: Workman Publishing, 2007), 199–200

58. Pamela Peeke, MD, *Fit to Live,* (New York: Rodale, Inc., 2007), pg. 155 and pg. 158.

59. Dorothy F. West, *Nutrition, Food, and Fitness* (Tinley Park: The Goodheart-Willcox Company, Inc., 2006), 256–261.

60. Mike Huckabee, *Quit Digging Your Grave with a Knife and Fork* (New York: Center Street—Time Warner Book Group, 2005), 62–63.

61. James M. Rippe, MD, *The Healthy Heart for Dummies* (Foster City: IDG Books Worldwide, 2000), pg. 67.

62. Michael F. Roizen, MD, *Real Age: Are You as Young as You Can Be?* (New York: Cliff Street Books—HarperCollins Publishers, 1999), pg. 207.

63. Robert K. Cooper, *Low-Fat Living* (Emmaus: Rodale Press, Inc., 1996, pg. 109.

64. Michael F. Roizen, MD, *Real Age: Are You as Young as You Can Be?* (New York: Cliff Street Books—HarperCollins Publishers, 1999), 213–216.

65. Chris Crowley and Henry Lodge, MD, *Younger Next Year* (New York: Workman Publishing, 2007), 66–67 and 79–80.

66. The psychological effects of exercise are experienced across the lifespan of children, adults, and older adults, by Michael R. Bracko, EdD, a fellow of the American College of Sports Medicine (ACSM).

67. A study published in 2007 by ACSM linked vigorous physical activity in kids to better grades in school by Bracko.

68. Kathleen Fackelmann, *Can't Remember What I Forgot: The Good News From the Front Lines of Memory Research* (New York: Harmony Books, 2008).

69. Pamela Peeke, MD, *Fit to Live* (New York: Rodale, Inc., 2007), pg. 168.

70. Robert K. Cooper, *Low-Fat Living* (Emmaus: Rodale Press, Inc. 1996), 100–101.

71. Howard Eisenson, MD, and Martin Binks, PhD, *The Duke Diet* (New York: Ballantine Books, 2007), pg. 61.

72. Mary Carmichael, "Stronger, Faster, Smarter," *Newsweek* (March 26, 2007): 38.

73. James M. Rippe, MD, *The Healthy Heart for Dummies* (Foster City: IDG Books Worldwide, 2000), pg. 8.

74. Robert K. Cooper, *Low-Fat Living* (Emmaus: Rodale Press, Inc., 1996), pg. 113.

75. Chris Crowley and Henry Lodge, MD, *Younger Next Year* (New York: Workman Publishing, 2007), pg. 64.

76. Chris Crowley and Henry Lodge, MD, *Younger Next Year* (New York: Workman Publishing, 2007), xxi.

77. Chris Crowley and Henry Lodge, MD, *Younger Next Year* (New York: Workman Publishing, 2007), pg. 64.

78. Chris Crowley and Henry Lodge, MD, *Younger Next Year* (New York: Workman Publishing, 2007), pg. 34 and pg. 52.

79. ConsumerReportsHealth.org experts, "10 Tips for a Healthy Heart," *Consumer Reports*, (May 2008): 40.

80. Zoe Elizabeth Buck, "It's Movement, Not Intensity that Matters," *Raleigh News & Observer*, published in the *Herald-Palladium*, (July 9, 2008).

81. Michael F. Roizen, MD, *The Real Age Makeover* (New York: HarperCollins, 2005), pg. 77 and pg. 323.

82. Dean Karnazes, *50/50: Secrets I Learned Running 50 Marathons in 50 Days—and How You Too Can Achieve Super Endurance*, (New York: Wellness Central, 2008), pg. 42.

83. Pamela Peeke, *Fit to Live* (New York: Rodale, Inc., 2007), 275–277.

84. Information from the U.S. Air Force Web site, containing exercise assessment tables and AFI 36–2905

85. (http://www.afpc.randolph.af.mil./shared/media/document/AFD-090820-144.pdf)

86. Deborah Kotz, "10 Healthy Habits That May Help You Live to 100," *U.S. News and World Report* (April 2009), references Thomas Perls, MD, MPH, Boston University School of Medicine, who studies the century-plus set.

Lightning Source UK Ltd.
Milton Keynes UK
UKOW03f0618130417
299019UK00001B/173/P

9 781449 079420